Rust Never Sleeps

by

Royce K. Bailey M.D., M.P.H.
Cardiologist

2012

Cover Design
Academy Press

Distributed by
Judy's Musical Ministry
50 Hospital Drive, Suite 3B
Hendersonville, NC 28792
(828) 684-2234
JudyWolterBailey.com

Contents

FORWARD

I have been blessed to work for Dr. Bailey for three years at the front desk of his office. One of my favorite times of the day is before we open, and Dr. Bailey comes by my window and we talk… we have shared laughter and tears – stories of his children, my grandchildren, mission work and music.

In the last two years I have helped with setting up and putting material on Park Ridge Cardiology's website (ParkRidgeCardiology.com) and reading and editing his Health Nuggets. I was very honored when Dr. Bailey asked me to write this Forward.

It's always great to see patients come out from an appointment with Dr. Bailey, so encouraged by his "alternative" ideas about their health concerns. He does prescribe traditional medicine as needed, but he tells them that there are also other ways to treat so many health issues, as he has experienced himself.

Our bodies are the temple of the Holy Spirit, as Scripture says in 1 Corinthians 6:19, and Dr. Bailey takes that very seriously as he encourages patients to look at all the things that are going on in their bodies, and then ask the Lord how best to begin the healing process. He continually writes articles and shares them with his patients on natural remedies and other medical things of interest he is finding out in his ongoing research.

I have been amazed to watch Dr. Bailey deal with his own physical health problems as a survivor of Crohn's Disease – actually with joy! – and out of that, learn to share with others the ways he has found to deal with what he is going through. He is an amazing man.

This book is a compilation of his latest Health Nuggets. It's definitely educational reading, but it's written in a fun, entertaining way. Look not only for health articles and recipes, but also devotional articles and information I encouraged him to include on delightful parenting techniques he and Judy used years ago. It's a book I recommend to all!

Of course, it's not done … Dr. Bailey continues to write. So stay tuned!!

Joyfully,
Marji Elzey
Park Ridge Cardiology

INTRODUCTION

I have been asked how I was able to find time to write on a variety of health subjects with a busy cardiology practice, home schooling our two daughters (now in college) and being the 'roadie' for my wife, Judy's, busy harp engagements around the country? First, you have to have very forgiving cardiology partners. Second, there is no time wasted. I don't play golf, and my hobbies are whatever the Bailey girls are doing, I'm doing too. I also read over six medical journals a week and glean new 'Health Nuggets' from them.

Back in the late 1990s I was asked by our church Sabbath School superintendent, Roberta Crabtree, to give a 5 minute health talk once a month called the 'Health Nugget.' I started out by just talking about a subject, but I couldn't keep to the 5 minute limit, so I started to write out what I was to say. Then people wanted copies, so I had to try and proof read the article and include my references. These added up over the years to my first book (2004), "You'll Rust Out Before You Wear Out, If...." Now I have compiled new or re-edited articles for a second book (2011), "Rust Never Sleeps." I want to thank Marji Elzey, Administrator of Front Office Management at Park Ridge Cardiology (ParkRidgeCardiology.com), for her editorial skills, proof reading and feed back.

So why call it "Rust Never Sleeps?" The inflammatory process in our body's arteries is constantly and chronically ongoing. By the Grace of God we don't all suddenly die of cancer, heart attacks and strokes. Our immune system must withstand incessant attacks every moment by bacteria, viruses, and mutated (cancer) cells. Therefore, we are slowly, day and night, rusting out as we age in this old world, but God has given us healthy alternatives to improve and extend our lives. Diet, exercise and a grateful heart are just the beginning of a new healthier you!

"The chief if not the only reason why many become invalids is that the blood does not circulate freely, and the changes in the vital fluid, which are necessary to life and health, do not take place. They have not given their bodies exercise nor their lungs food, which is pure, fresh air; therefore it is impossible for the blood to be vitalized, and it pursues its course sluggishly through the system. The more we exercise, the better will be the circulation of the blood. ***More people die for want of exercise than through over fatigue; very many more rust out than wear out.*** *Those who accustom themselves to proper exercise in the open air will generally have a good and vigorous circulation. We are more dependent upon the air we breathe than upon the food we eat. Men and women,*

young and old, who desire health, and who would enjoy active life, should remember that they cannot have these without a good circulation. Whatever their business and inclinations, they should make up their minds to exercise in the open air as much as they can. They should feel it a religious duty to overcome the conditions of health which have kept them confined indoors, deprived of exercise in the open air." Ellen G. White, Testimonies For The Church, Vol. 2; 1870:525-6.

THE GREAT AMERICAN DIET

- Always Tired - Thin Bones - No Energy - Too Many Combinations?

Part 1
Metabolic Syndrome X

Over half of the people in the United States have Metabolic Syndrome X. It will shorten your life! Are you prediabetic?

Fast food came to the Cherokee Indian Reservation, NC in 1982. Now diabetes is affecting younger and younger people on the reservation. The shift from game and a whole foods-based diet to one of convenience has disastrous effects.

Seeing what people eat in the Great American Diet is the tip of the iceberg to the problem.

-Eat more protein? -Eat more calcium? -Eat more sugar? So we get osteoporosis, heart disease, diabetes, cancer, early aging, and we're always tired. The Great American Diet is nutritionally impoverished from empty calories, low fiber, high fat and sugar diets. No wonder that so many of us are OVERFED and UNDERNOURISHED. This is a "McDonald's" type diet. This is the Great American Diet.

Metabolic Syndrome X is therefore made up of the deadly quartet of high triglycerides, central obesity, hypertension and hyperinsulinemia (high fasting blood sugars). This includes dense small LDL (bad cholesterol), low HDL (good cholesterol) and hyper-coagulability (makes clots/scabs in the blood vessels easily).

Your Acid/Base Balance

pH is the electrical balance between negative hydroxyl (OH-) ions (alkalinity) compared to positive hydrogen (H+) ions (acidity). The pH scale runs from 0 (most acidic) to 14 (most alkaline). To survive, our bodies must stay on the alkaline side of neutral pH 7.4. It takes vital force to stay alkaline. If you become too acidic for whatever reason, you will develop disease or die. Long distance runners can have severe fatigue, muscle failure and cramping, because muscle waste products are acidic (Lactic Acidosis). Our Great American Diet causes us to be more acidic! Most foods are either acid or alkaline producing. Scientists have known for over 100 years that by simply changing one's diet you could change the body's pH. Bringing your pH closer to normal helps the sick get rid of many of their health complaints. Unfortunately, mainstream medicine has never fully accepted this concept.

Our Vanishing Bones And Muscles

Doctors' recommendation for thin bones is to increase your calcium intake, which never has been shown to make much difference. So it's up to you! If your pH drops to 7.38, the body breaks down bone and muscle to neutralize the acid. Your bones are the body's ultimate acid neutralizing storage facility. 25% to 30% of all nursing home patients are there because of a hip fracture. The rate of hip fractures has doubled in the last 50 years (corrected for the increased elderly in our population). There are over 2.3 million hip fractures a year, worldwide. One in every six Americans will suffer a hip fracture (30% are men). Why? --Osteoporosis (thin bones). Acidic pH destroys living bone. Add to that our lack of Vitamin D and exercise. No wonder our bones break at such a high rate!

Our gradual muscle loss from chronic acidosis is first noticed with weakness in the thighs and legs. It is hard to get out of a chair or car and harder to walk without help. Exercise will temporarily help, but without changing to a more alkaline producing diet the overall benefit will be marginal.

Sources Of Acid Disposal

Your blood is one of the primary means for removal of the body's acidic waste products. Blood carries acid to your kidneys. Carbonic acid is carried to your lungs and released as CO_2 and H_2O. Your liver and pancreas make alkaline enzymes to help reduce excess acidity. Lymphatic tissue (Peyer's patches) in the small bowel produce large amounts of alkalizing enzymes called chyle. Sweat glands and evacuation from the large bowel also help lower the body's acid load. But in Western Society that is not enough alkali to neutralize all the acid!

Bone Loss And Your Acid Producing Diet

A review of 85 studies in 33 countries found that diets high in animal protein (fish, meat and cheese) have a direct relationship to the incidence of hip fractures. Germany and Sweden had 40 times as many hip fractures as did Thailand. Women eating a high acid-producing diet had a more rapid bone loss and a 3.7 times greater risk of hip fracture than women eating a neutral or alkaline producing diet.

What's Wrong With Cheese?

Milk contains equal parts acid and alkaline producing compounds. Remember the nursery rhyme, "Little Miss Muffet, sat on her tuffet, eating her curds and way (whey)." Acidic casein (curds) and alkaline whey are the two parts. In cheese production the liquid alkaline whey portion is removed, therefore, the more sharp or crumbly the cheese the more acidic it is. Parmesan cheese is the most acid forming. It can take the body hours up to three days to correct the body acid condition cheese leaves in your tissues. Ripened (dry/hard) "cheese should never be introduced into the stomach."[2]

Don't Oxidize The Butter

"Butter is less harmful when eaten on cold bread than when used in cooking."[3] Butter oxidizes when left out for as little as 20 minutes and oxidizes when heated. Oxidation is a toxic (rusting) process involving the bad cholesterol-LDL, which causes damage to the blood vessel walls, increasing the risk of heart attacks and strokes.

Does Protein Cause Bone Loss?

Not all proteins are created equal. Animal proteins are strong acid-forming foods, whereas vegetable proteins contain enough alkaline compounds to neutralize any acidic effects. This would explain some of the confusing findings about high protein diets causing or not causing bone loss. It depends on the protein source. This is just one of the reasons I don't recommend an Atkins (high protein) diet.

I Hate Vegetables

My middle brother (PhD) is a pastor in Texas and has never, since he was a baby, liked vegetables. My brother's excuse is, *"But I don't like vegetables, because they were made to eat after sin."* Gen. 3:18 Fruits and vegetables contain about the same vitamins and minerals, but vegetables offer a wider array of compounds that protect from cancer and heart disease. Broccoli and other cruciferous vegetables, but not a single fruit, are packed with sulphoraphane, which fight cancers, including breast cancer.

Stomach Acid

The stomach's parietal cells secrete an acid solution that contains 160 millimoles of hydrochloric acid per liter. The pH of this acid is about 0.8, (your body pH is 7.4) demonstrating its extreme acidity. To concentrate the hydrogen ions this much requires more than 1500 calories of energy per liter of gastric juice. At this pH, the hydrogen ion concentration is about 3 million times that of the arterial blood, but is isotonic with the body fluids. The total gastric juice secretion (it is not all hydrochloric acid) is about 1 1/2 liters per day. By eating a combination of foods at the same meal (mixing fruits and vegetables at one meal), it will make your body and blood stream hypertonic and more acidic.

Don't Mix Your Fruits And Veggies

I recommend 9 pieces of fruit or vegetables a day, but don't eat them at the same meal. The reason is that fruits and vegetables eaten together at one meal produce hyper-acidity of the blood stream. This requires neutralization by your bicarbonate buffer reserves (like an alkali bank account) which take vital force. The right alkaline balance of the blood is maintained by foods, kidneys, pores, lungs (which eliminate acids) and your buffer system. Consequently, if a hyper acidic state occurred day after day, year in and year out, it could shorten your life. When the alkalies in your body are deficient, life ceases; and when the acids are in excess, life ceases.

Understanding of this simple chemistry of our bodies makes it very plain that foods and food combinations will influence our bodies on a daily basis. Our mood, our closeness to God, or our rebelliousness and our very personality will be affected.

Footnotes:

1. We're told to avoid the sun because of the potential for skin cancer, but our high fat diets are frying our skin. We need at least 15 minutes of sunshine a day.
2. White, E.G., Testimonies To The Church, Vol 2;1868:68
3. White, E.G., Ministry of Health;1905:302.

Part 2

Food lovers believe that eating is one of life's greatest pleasures. But if they could only see that it can become one of life's greatest causes of misery.

Fermentation Causes Acidosis

Raw fruits and raw veggies require totally different enzyme combinations for their effective digestion. Your body faces a dilemma: it will try to digest the vegetables first and the fruit, which requires no stomach digestion is held up and will start to ferment (producing unwanted acidosis), thus further delaying digestion. This process will ultimately deliver contaminants to your blood stream. Other factors that retard proper digestion and thus increase the likelihood of causing fermentation include: baking soda, condiments of all kinds (which either destroy the enzymes or inhibit secretion of digestive juices), salt (in any quantity greater than a small amount) and eating complex mixtures of foods. Simplify your diet. The simpler the better! Your food should be as close to the way it comes from the garden for the best results. I personally can tell a difference when I get too many combinations in how I feel, my mood, my sleep patterns and my energy level.

Too Many Combinations

I have patients that tell me that they don't notice any increased gas, brain fog or indigestion when they eat a large amount of combinations including fruits and vegetables. That's because they are eating so many combinations of foods that their bodies are always acidic and feeding their blood stream partially digested nutrients. They are so used to feeling this way; they don't know the best they can feel.

There is one exception to this rule of not combining fruits and vegetables; you may combine acid citrus fruits, pineapple, papaya and avocado, for example, with your veggies. This is because these are alkaline forming in your body. So it is best to avoid acid producing starchy vegetables with your fruits, like: corn, potatoes, sweet potatoes, yams, winter squashes, such as pumpkin, butternut squash, acorn squash, dried beans, peas and lentils.

The Real Acid Forming Foods

When I talk about certain foods being acid foods (like lemons, oranges, strawberries, cherries, etc.), I do not mean they are acid-forming in the body. These fruits actually are alkaline in reaction to the body after they are eaten, provided the alkaline reserve (bicarbonate buffer) is high enough to convert the acid. My patients that cannot eat citrus, because it burns their stomach, usually will be found to have a very acidic body pH. Changing their diet to an alkaline based diet will resolve their acidic complaints. Acidic foods that are alkaline producing in your body, burned as fuel in the cells, produce energy and make carbonic acid gas, which is shuttled by the lymph and blood to the lungs and exhaled. About 30 quarts of carbonic acid gas (about a third of all body wastes) are exhaled per hour by the average individual, leaving the body no harm and in an alkali state.

The real acid forming foods have a lot of starch, protein and fat in them; beans, nuts, eggs, meats and cheese. Foods that are acid or alkaline forming depend on how they are cooked and eaten. For example, a mealy baked potato is alkaline in reaction if it is chewed well, and if the skins are eaten. If it is washed down or swallowed whole, the digestion is not complete, and it is acid-forming. Similarly, putting sour cream on that same potato or frying it, making it greasy, makes it acid forming.

What's The Remedy For Too Much Acid?

Long before dialysis for kidney failure, doctors knew to give bicarbonate of soda (baking soda) to relieve bloated stomachs. They found that these patients' bones began to re-mineralize and get stronger. Even today I will add sodium bicarbonate tabs 600 mg three times a day for renal failure patients to balance their insufficient excretion of acid from the kidneys. Many studies have been done to evaluate this acid/base effect. Many people take bicarbonates at mealtime, but this neutralizes the stomach acid needed to digest their food. They are just treating the symptoms (an overly acid diet), not the problem! Eating an acid producing diet may not have caused you any problems yet, but eventually you'll pay with your health. The NO-BRAINER is to change your diet to an alkaline based diet. Duh!

Desert the dessert. Eaten on top of meals, desserts lie heavy on the stomach, fermenting and slowing the total digestive process down. Bacteria turns desserts into alcohols, vinegars and acetic acid.

Are You Suffocating?

Poor oxygen utilization originates from acidosis. I studied this oxygen saturation curve in medical school. One of the primary waste products of the body is carbon dioxide (CO_2). Alkaline compounds (bicarbonates) are required in your cells to exchange oxygen for CO_2. When your alkali supply is too low, CO_2 stays in the cells and piles up in the suffocating tissues. "The Great American Diet" causes chronic acidosis which causes "couch potato" people to sigh a lot, experience breathlessness, pant at the least exertion, have frequent muscle pain, have insomnia (can't sleep), have a constant "lump" in their throat (from dehydration and loss of sodium), have chronic fatigue, have blisters in their mouth from eating citrus, have low back pain, have recurrent urinary tract infections, have symptomatic low blood pressures and have difficulty holding their breath for at least 20 seconds. If you have any of these symptoms you probably are too acidic.

Starving For Air?

In scuba diving, divers that are more acidic run out of air quickly; while those that are more pH balanced can make a tank of air "last forever." A blood gas analysis from your artery is the best way to check your pH, but you may also check your saliva, because it approximates the blood pH at 6.5 to 7.0. If your saliva consistently falls below 6.5, you are too acidic. If yours consistently reads above 7.0, you could be too alkaline. You can find test strips on the internet. Urine tests aren't accurate for body pH.

Acidosis-Cancer, Diabetes And Heart Disease

Acidic abundance in your tissue is common during the initial formation of cancer. Hyper acidity appears to contribute to insulin sensitivity problems that lead to diabetes. Chronic acidosis is underlying in the number one killer: heart disease. Acidosis interferes with the exchange of oxygen and CO2 at the cellular level, suffocating the heart muscle, causing the heart to pump harder and more often to supply oxygen to the other organs of the body. The natural ratio for a healthy body is four parts alkaline to one part acid (ratio 4:1). When such a ratio is maintained, the body has a strong resistance against disease. Remember, alkali bases neutralize acids. It is just as dangerous to become too alkaline as too acidic; temperance in all things.

So What Can I Do?

The first adjustment is to eat a more alkaline diet, not mix fruits and vegetables (because you are eating more simply, you will notice) and 50% - 85% of your food should be raw (i.e., fruits and veggies). When this is done, there will be little to no room for meat, fish, or fowl. You need 75-80% of your food to be alkaline. If you are not eating a diet rich in whole grains, fruits and veggies, you're not getting enough base containing foods. Vegetable juicing can jump-start this process of alkalinizing your body. If you make these changes in your diet you can experience a dramatic difference in your health in just a couple of weeks.

I'm So Tired!

Weariness comes from these acid-forming wastes in your body. The custom of the day is to eat a highly acid diet and we wonder why we are so chronically fatigued and can't sleep at night! The tiredness from which one can not rest, the inability to concentrate on mental work or to apply one's self to the day's task is, in many cases, from poisoning of the nerve cells. This is because of the pollution of the body fluids which bathe all those vital cells. In the lab, nerves can't be fatigued when repeatedly stimulated, but the accumulation and over-production of acid products "drugs" the nerves, ultimately injuring them, sometimes permanently.

We Need Less Protein

If you follow this counsel you will need much less protein in your diet. This is the second adjustment. Due to an acid medium's rapid destruction of protein, the body's requirement for protein increases, while an alkaline environment spares this usual destruction of protein. Eating less protein will protect your kidneys and extend your life. When I speak of protein most people think of meat, which is very concentrated. Don't do as so many before have done and substitute eggs and bread for meat, or sugar for meat; all of which are acid forming. If you do this, you have made the problem worse.

Stuff We Should Have Known!

"There should not be a great variety at any one meal, for this encourages overeating and causes indigestion."

"It is not well to eat fruit and vegetables at the same meal. If digestion is feeble, the use of both will often cause distress, and inability to put forth mental effort. It is better to have fruit at one meal, and the vegetables at another." 1905

"Many are made sick by indulgence of their appetite... So many varieties are introduced into the stomach that fermentation is the result. This condition brings on acute disease, and death frequently follows." 1897

"If your work is sedentary, take exercise every day and at each meal eat two or three kinds of simple food taking no more of these than will satisfy the demands of hunger." 1896

"Disturbance is created by improper combinations of food; fermentation sets in; the blood is contaminated and the brain confused... In vain the stomach protests, and appeals to the brain to reason from cause to effect. The excessive amount of food eaten, or the improper combination, does its injurious work" 1902

"Many eat too rapidly. Others eat at one meal food which does not agree. If men and women would only remember how greatly they afflict the soul when they afflict the stomach, and how deeply Christ is dishonored when the stomach is abused, they would be brave and self denying, giving the stomach opportunity to recover its healthy action. While sitting at the table we may do medical missionary work by eating and drinking to the Glory of God." 1901

"The digestive organs have an important part to act in our life happiness. God has given us intelligence, that we may learn what we should use as food. Shall we not, as sensible men and women, study whether the things we eat will be in agreement, or whether they will cause trouble? People who have a sour stomach are very often of a sour disposition. Everything seems to be contrary to them, and they are inclined to be peevish and irritable. If we would have peace among

ourselves, we should give more thought than we do to having a peaceful stomach." 1908

"I took notice of your diet. You eat too great a variety at one meal. Fruit and vegetables taken at one meal produce acidity of the stomach; then impurity of the blood results, and the mind is not clear because the digestion is imperfect." 1908

4. Because of the problem with sugar loads, just juice vegetables, not fruits.

References:

Williams, D, *"Getting Back To Our Roots,"* Alternatives, May 2002; 9(11):81-88.
Sebastian, A .J., Genontology Annals Biol Sci & Med Sci, 2000; P55(10):M585-92.
Sellmeyer, D., AmJ Clin Nutr, 2001;74(3):41 1-412.
Sebastian, A. J., N Engl J Med, 1994;330(25):1776-81. Similar studies: Kidney Int, 1989;35:688-95; Israel J Med Sci, 1971;7:499; Am J Clin Nutr, 1984; 39:281-88.
Remer, T.Z., Ernahrungswiss, 1995;34(1):10-15. Research Institute of Child Nutrition, Dortrnund, Germany.
Sebastian, A. J., Am J Clin Nutr, 2001;73(1):118-122.
Moore, C., *"Fruit Alone Doesn't Cut It,"* www.Prevention.com, Sept. 2000; 82.
Paulien, G.B., *"The Divine Philosophy And Science Of Health And 63 Healing,"* Teach Services, Inc, 1995;124,129-132.
Guyton, A., *"Textbook Of Medical Physiology",* WB Saunders Co., 9th ed., 1994; 819-820.
Shelton, H.M., *"Exercise",* Natural Hygiene Press, Chicago, IL., 1971.
White, G.J., *"Abundant Heath",* Health and Character Education Institute, 1951; 43-59.
White, E.G., *"Counsels on Diet and Foods,"* Pacific Press Pub. Ass., 1938;110-113.

ACID BASED FOODS

There are varying degrees of acidity in our foods; the more natural the better, the more processed the worst. I have found multiple lists, not all the same, containing acid and alkaline foods. This outline is a mix of many lists and may not match up exactly to your list.

Acid Forming Foods

All meats (beef, pork, chicken) and fish
Cheese, along with sharper/dry cheeses (with Parmesan the worst)
Colas (phosphorus in colas turns to phosphoric acid and destroys bone)
Alcohol
Caffeinated drinks, coffee
Sweetened yogurt
Artificial sweeteners, processed cane and beet sugar, barley syrup, heat processed honey (cold extracted is alkaline), maple sugar, molasses, fructose, lactose, refined table sugar

Anything fried or barbecued
Soy sauce
Mustard (dried and processed)
Ketchup (unless natural and homemade without vinegar)
Apple cider, sweet brown rice vinegar, white vinegar
Nutmeg
Tobacco
Practically all prescription drugs

Mildly Acid Forming Or Neutral

Sunflower and pumpkin seeds
Wheat germ
Nuts, including walnuts, pecans, cashews, dried coconut (fresh is alkaline), pistachios, macadamias, filberts, peanuts
Rice (white, brown and basmati)
Cornmeal, oats, rye, spelt, wheat, bran
Popcorn
Pastas
Breads and most other grain products like cereals (hot or cold), crackers, pastries
The following beans (unless sprouted which makes them alkaline): pinto, navy, mung, lentils, black, garbanzo, red, white, adzuki, broad

Alkalizing Foods

Practically all vegetables
Practically all fruits, except blueberries, plums, prunes, cranberries. Even citrus such as lemons, which many think of as being acidic, are alkaline producing in the body. They are rich in organic salts, like citrates, which are converted into bicarbonates.
Beans, like string, soy, lima, green, snap Peas Potatoes (not fried)
Arrowroot flour grains, like flax, millet, quinoa, amaranth
Nuts, like almonds, pignoli (pine nut), chestnuts, Brazil nuts
Sprouted anything, including alfalfa, radish, chia
Unsprouted, untoasted seeds, like sesame
Fresh unsalted buttermilk and cream Goat's milk
Eggs
Whey
Plain yogurt
Sweeteners, like raw, unpasteurized honey, dried sugar cane juice (sucanat), brown rice syrup

Fruit juices
All vegetable juices
Most herbal teas
Garlic
Cayenne pepper
Almost all herbs
Miso
Most vegetable and unprocessed sea salt
Almost all spices
Vanilla extract
Brewer's or nutritional yeast
Most unprocessed, cold-pressed oils are neutral or alkaline forming (even margarine, but I would avoid this "liquid plastic")

'BONE' APPETITE

- Your Bones Are What You Eat
- Controversies In Calcium
- What Makes Strong Bones For Life?

Requirements For Calcium Absorption

Calcium is the most abundant mineral in the body. Every cell requires calcium. Most chemical reactions in your body require calcium. 99% of your body's calcium stores are in your bones and teeth. Calcium is essential for proper blood clotting, nerve impulse function, muscle operation and proper bone, teeth and cartilage formation. Proper calcium absorption requires vitamins A, D, C, phosphorus, boron and magnesium. Note, fluoride is not needed for absorption.

Bone Loss

Bone loss is not just a old age problem. You start to lose calcium bone mass at around age 35. Most women have 22 pounds of calcium in their body, but by age 45 they have lost 2 pounds of bone. By age 55, they have lost another four pounds. At age 60 the average American female has lost another three pounds of bone. That's almost 40% of your bone mass lost before you even reach retirement age!

What Causes Calcium Loss?

We all should be protecting our calcium stores. Once calcium is lost it is very hard to restore it to near-normal. If there is not enough calcium in your diet where does your body get extra calcium? If there is not enough calcium in your blood stream where does your body get extra calcium? What causes calcium loss? Your diet!!! Lifestyle causes osteoporosis (thin bones):

- Lack of weight bearing exercises. Astronauts lose 200 mg/d of calcium in space.
- Excess protein intake. (> 65 grams/day, recommended .8 gm/kg)
- Caffeine intake.
- Nicotine.
- Carbonated beverages.
- Lack of sun exposure.
- Excess salt

But I Want My Soda

Calcium (Ca) binds with phosphorus roughly one to one. In a simplified explanation of the chemistry, high phosphorus (high salt/protein) diets (soft drinks are high in phosphoric acid) are usually two phosphorus molecules to one calcium molecule. Again, where does the body get the extra calcium to bind the outstanding phosphorus? From the blood stream. What if it is not available in the blood stream? It steals the extra calcium from your bones. What happens when your bones are finally depleted?

Deficiencies Are Not Seen In Third World Countries

It was found that African women over 60 years old who rarely, if ever, ate dairy products, consumed only 250-400 mg of calcium a day from vegetables and had an average of ten children in their life, had healthy bones and no calcium deficiency. But young women eating the Great American Diet (McDonald's type) who had no children, were eating heavily of dairy products and consuming over 500 mg of calcium/day, suffered significant loses of calcium from their bones. Native women who moved to the city and began eating the Great American Diet, suffered significant loses of calcium from both their bones and teeth. Research shows that the National Institutes of Health Recommended Daily Allowance (RDA) of 1500 mg of calcium a day isn't even enough for those who eat the Great American Diet! Why?

Brain-Washed By The Milk Board

But milk is good for your bones-RIGHT? The Milk Board (The

United States Lobby For Milk Use) would have you think so. Milk is touted as preventing osteoporosis, yet clinical research shows otherwise. The Harvard Nurses Health Study, followed 75,000 women for 12 years, showed that a increased intake of calcium from dairy products was associated with a higher fracture risk. Do you remember the Ad, "Everybody Needs Milk?" In 1974, the Federal Trade Commission found the Milk Ad Campaign deceptive. Several very large studies showed excellent absorption of calcium from milk into the blood stream, but did not demonstrate increased bone calcium mass. Later smaller studies showed that the higher the protein content in the diet, the more calcium was lost through the kidneys, with a net total loss of body calcium when milk was consumed.

Eat Your Protein, Lose Your Bones

The higher the protein in the diet the better-RIGHT? Unprocessed plant-based foods easily meet the protein needs for both adults and children. But no study exists proving that high blood level of calcium from milk and meat ended up in your bones. In fact, the higher the daily protein intake, (and milk is a protein and acts like a solid in your stomach), the less calcium was found in the bones. Why? Milk is made up of two parts 1. Casein (Curds) 2. Whey Remember "Little Miss Muffit sat on a tuffit eating her curds and whey." Casein acts like a diuretic of calcium. The more casein eaten the more wasting of calcium in your urine. Also, the more protein eaten, the more wasting of calcium in your urine. So, milk can cause a double calcium loss; ultimately thinning your bones.

The Long-Term Problem With High Protein

Quick weight loss programs emphasizing high protein diets include: Atkins, Zone, Protein Power, Sugar Busters and the Stillman Diet. These diets are rich in protein and animal/saturated fat, such as meat, meat substitutes, cheese, milk and eggs. Long-term diets high in fatty animal foods increase your risk for: coronary artery disease, diabetes, stroke, cancer, compromised vitamin and mineral intake, worsened liver and kidney disease. Here are some reasons for high protein diets: They may provide a quick drop in weight; this is through the loss of fluid, by the diuretic effect of eliminating too many carbohydrates; Complex carbohydrates reduce blood pressure and cholesterol, but replacing them, however, raises bad oxidized Cholesterol (LDL). My patients say this is the only way they have been able to lower their blood sugar and lose weight. But it doesn't last for long. No one can live on eight eggs a day for long. There is a healthier way.

Magnesium (Mg) Deficiency

We've tilled our soil for 200 years. Most of our fresh fruits/veggies in the winter come from outside the United States, and they have tilled their soil for over 2000 years. Our calcium ratio should be two calcium molecules to every one magnesium molecule (2:1). The usual American diet with calcium supplements of 1500mg/day is a five calcium to one magnesium ratio (5:1). Intakes and nutrients that increase magnesium need in the body include: fats, calcium, phosphate, Vitamin D, sugar, alcohol, high fiber (interferes with mineral absorption) and Cortisone (Prednisone) Calcium/Magnesium Deficiency and Stroke.

Finland has the highest stroke and ischemic heart disease rate in the world for young and middle aged men. Finland follows the Great American Diet: low fiber, high sugar, high salt, high protein, 50% empty calorie diet (Junk Food). Finland has a life long Ca/Mg ratio of 4:1. Osteoporosis is prevalent. Japan has the best Ca/Mg ratio of all industrialized countries. Japan has the lowest heart disease when not adopting a Western Diet. Magnesium is an essential part of the organic bone matrix. Calcium supplements intensify the negative Mg balances in your body.

Long-Term Magnesium Deficiency Cause:

- Arrhythmias (High Mg < Adrenaline release)
- Sudden Death
- Vascular damage, i.e. Arteriosclerosis
- Hypertension (Free intracellular Mg is depressed)
- Kidney stones
- Brittle bones
- Hypercoagulability (can make blood clots)
- Eclampsia
- Calcinosis (Calcium in soft-tissue other than bone)

Magnesium Deficiency May Lead To:

- Irritability
- Mental fog
- Muscle weakness
- Cramping
- Palpitations
- Low potassium levels

Which Kind Of Calcium?

Calcium is an unstable mineral. In nature it is almost always found as a calcium salt. Like calcium plus carbon (carbonate), calcium plus citric acid (citrate), calcium plus lactate (found in milk) and calcium plus animal bone (hydroxyapatite).

The vast majority of calcium sold in the stores is calcium carbonate (including coral calcium and antacids like Tums). It's cheap and plentiful, but absorption into our bones is only about 20%, so you have to take a lot. The fracture rate for those taking calcium carbonate is still 357 fractures/ one thousand patient years in one study. Calcium citrate is easily absorbed but contains only 10% elemental calcium. That's why calcium citrate pills are so large.

The best source of calcium is from vegan sources. There may not be very much calcium in these sources but all of this calcium goes to your bones: Tofu, Rhubarb, Collard greens, Spinach, Turnip greens, Okra, White beans, Baked beans, Broccoli, Peas, Brussel sprouts, Sesame seeds, Bok choy, Dried fruit, Brazil nuts and Almonds (six almonds/day gives 84mg magnesium and 75 mg of calcium).

Boron

Boron is the forgotten trace mineral. Boron influences Ca and Mg metabolism to prevent bone demineralization. Boron helps cell membrane function. It increases concentrations of plasma estrogen and decreases cardiovascular disease incidence. Boron assists in the development of new bone.

What Do You Know About Vitamin D?

A recent study found that 57% of the people admitted to a Boston Hospital had a Vitamin D deficiency. Sunlight on unprotected skin causes the body to produce vitamin D. Get 15 minutes of sunshine a day on your hands, feet, back of your legs and arms. If your bones are thin consider taking 5000 International Units of Vitamin D a day to make up for your lack of sun exposure.

Vitamin D deficiency:

- Decreases bone mass.
- Increases risk of fractures.
- Increases risk of kidney stones.
- Causes muscle weakness.
- Worsens generalized fibromyalgia-type pain and peripheral neuropathy.
- Worsens Multiple Sclerosis (MS).

- May contribute to autism.
- Increases risk of many cancers.
- May induce diabetes.
- Increases risk of vascular disease and hypertension.
- Worsens Polycytic Ovarian Syndrome (PCOS).
- Worsens depression.
- Worsens balance problems and causes more falls.

Vitamin K

Vitamin K helps prevent arterial calcifications (hardening of the arteries) by keeping the calcium in your bones, not in your tissues. Calcium supplements alone can be detrimental and then can seep into your arteries. Imagine a vitamin that could keep calcium in bones and out of your arteries. Vitamin K is found in abundance in green veggies. Avoid Vitamin K if you are taking Coumadin/Warfarin, for it attaches to the same clotting receptor as coumadin, thus making your blood too thick.

Calcium Study

If you have had a bone density study and have found your bone too thin, here are my recommendations for stronger bones:

- Calcium/Magnesium supplement with a ratio of 2:1 (like 1500 mg Ca/750 mg Mg)
- Vitamin D (sun and pill 5000 IU)
- Boron 3 mg/day
- Avoid high protein and salt diets
- Vitamin K 5-10 mg/day
- One ounce of water for every kilogram of your body weight every day
- Daily exercise
- An alkaline diet (fruits, nuts, grains, veggies) vs. the Great "Acidic" American Diet
- *"A merry heart doeth good like a medicine, but a broken spirit drieth the bones "* Proverbs 17:22

References:

Lovendale, M., *"Are Cows Hurting Children?"* Quality Longevity.

Walker, *"Calcium Study,"* Clinical Science, 1972.

Anad, C., *"Effects of Protein Intake on Calcium Balance of Young Men Given 500mg Calcium Daily,"* Journal of Nutrition, 1974;104:695.

Feshanich, D., *"Milk, Dietary Calcium, And Bone Fractures In Women: A 12-year Prospective Study,"* Am J Public Health, 1997;87:992-7.

Oski, F., *"Don't Drink Your Milk,"* Mollica Press, LTD, Syracuse, NY; 1983.

Nomilk.com and Notmilk.com are good resources.

Hegstead, M. *"Urinary Calcium and Calcium Balance in Young Men as Affected by Level of Protein and Phosphorous Intake."* Journal of Nutrition, 1981;111:53.

Finn, S.C., *"The Skeleton Crew: Is Calcium Enough?"* J Women Health, 1998;7(1):31-6.

USDA, *"Bone Loss, Phosphorous And Soft Drinks,"* Nutrition Week, September 18, 1998;28(36):7

Walker, R., *"Calcium Retention In The Adult Human Male As Affected By Protein Intake,"* Journal of Nutrition, 1972;102:1297.

Johnson, N., *"Effect of Level of Protein Intake on Urinary and Fecal Calcium and Calcium Retention of Young Adult Males,"* Journal of Nutrition, 1970;100:1425.

Linkswiler, H., *"Calcium Retention of Young Adults Males As Affected by Level of Protein and Calcium Intake,"* Trans New York Academy of Science, 1974;38:333.

McDougal, J., *"McDougal's Medicine,"* New Publishers, NY, 1985.

Karppanen, H., *"Magnesium Bulletin,"* 1990;12:80-86.

Seelig, M.S., *"Magnesium Deficiency In The Pathogenesis Of Disease. Early Roots of Cardiovascular, Skeletal, and Renal Abnormalities."* Publ Plenum Press, NY, 1980.

Thomas M., "Vitamin D Deficiency Is Very Common," Harvard Medical School News Letter, 5/1/02.

Hunt, C.D., *"Metabolic Responses Of Postmenopausal Women To Supplemental Dietary Boron and Aluminum, During Usual And Low Magnesium Intake: Boron, Calcium, And Magnesium Absorption And Retention And Blood Mineral Concentration,"* Am J Clin Nutr, 1997;65:803-813.

Samman, S., *"Minor Dietary Factors In Relation To Coronary Heart Disease-Flavonoids, Isoflavones And Boron,"* J Clin Biochem Nutr, 1996;20:173-180.

Vitamin K Articles:

Circulation 2000,102:380-385

J Am Col Card 2000;36(1):326-340

Hematol Oncol Clin North Am 2000 Apr;14(2):339-353

Int J Exp Pathol 2000 Feb;81(1):51-56

Tucker, K.L., *"Potassium, Magnesium, And Fruit And Vegetable Intakes Are Associated With Greater Bone Mineral Density In Elderly Men And Women,"* Am J Clin Nutr, 1999;69:727-36.

VINEGAR TOO?

- Avoiding this Acid Will Improve Your Health
- Vinegar Worsens Heartburn

The name VINEGAR comes from the simple compounding of two words by the French, probably not uttered pleasantly. When a cask of wine got a crack in it and became exposed to air, they most likely uttered ......vin ..aiger ....which means ..sour wine. So how does this work? First the sugars from the fruit (usually grapes or apples/cider) must change to alcohol. Then airborne (aerobic) bacteria turn the alcohol into acetic acid.

What To Do About Our Love Of A Tart Taste

But I've changed, you say, so many of my 'favorite' destructive dietary habits to be healthier and now you want me to give up using vinegar too? You must read the labels; vinegar is in more than you may think. Vinegar is an ingredient in many prepared foods, from salad dressings and baked beans, to pickles, green stuffed olives and even some commercial breads. Meals are more satisfying and enjoyable when they include a variety of flavors, including tart flavors, but these should come from natural, wholesome tart foods. Naturally tart foods would include lemons and limes. Citrus, though acid to the taste, metabolize to an alkaline ash in the human body; so citrus actually increases the alkaline reserve of the blood, rather than reducing it as vinegar does. Lemon or lime juice is excellent on salads, much better than vinegar. Lemon or lime juice may be used in the preparation of most foods, such as baked beans, where vinegar was used in the past. Orange segments or juice may be added for the sweet/sour effect, and a little of the grated rind (zest) may be added for extra flavor and nutrients.

Too Acidic

Some of my patients say they cannot eat citrus because it worsens their heartburn. This is because their body's acid/base balance is so far out of balance (too acidic). They will be able to eat citrus once again if they eat a plant based alkaline diet daily and avoid acid producing fried, low fiber, high sugar, high carbs Great American type diet.

So why is vinegar so bad?

Prevents The Break Down Of Carbohydrates

"Vinegar contains acetic acid. The same fermentation process by which alcohol is produced results in acetic acid when the process is carried a little farther. Vinegar is much more irritating to the digestive organs than an alcoholic liquor of the same strength. Even in a small quantity it completely prevents the action of saliva on starch." J.H.Kellogg, "The Home Book of Modern Medicine," 1893:289.

Prevents The Break Down Of Protein

"Vinegar also lowers the alkaline reserve of the blood, is said to aid in destroying red blood cells, hinders the digestion of protein, and is an active agent in the liver damage (cirrhosis)." Julius Gilbert White, "Abundant Health," 1932:131. A lack of an alkaline reserve causes osteoporosis (thin breakable bones). Acidic vinegar worsens heart burn and reflux symptoms.

Fermentation Causes Impurities

"The salads are prepared with oil and vinegar, fermentation takes place in the stomach, and the food does not digest, but decays or

putrefies; as a consequence, the blood is not nourished, but becomes filled with impurities, and the liver and kidney difficulties appear." Ellen G. White, "Counsels On Diet And Foods," 345.

Why Have Vinegar In Your House?

Buying distilled vinegar in a gallon bottle is very economical. It cleans, deodorizes and sanitizes almost as well or better than anything on the market.

- It is a natural way to get rid of ants and other insects.
- It kills unwanted bacteria such as E Coli. Michael Mullen a spokesperson for the Heinz Corporation says that straight 5% vinegar will kill 80% of the germs and viruses in your house. Heinz says they can't make the claim on the bottle that it kills bacteria because of the EPA laws.
- Toothbrushes can be boiled for a minute in vinegar to kill the germs.
- Vinegar relieves itching from mosquito or bug bites, soothes sunburn pains and jelly fish stings.
- Keeping a spray bottle of straight 5% distilled vinegar is useful to clean, disinfect and sanitize many things like your cutting board, microwave or refrigerator. Place 1 cup of apple cider vinegar in a glass and set it in your refrigerator. Within 2 days, any smell will be gone!
- Try spraying vinegar on hard to clean kitchen appliances that have many nooks and crannies, that come in contact with bacteria. Spray it on door handles, and all the bathroom fixtures to disinfect them.
- To kill grass or weeds on sidewalks and driveways, spray full strength white distilled vinegar on it.
- You can also kill molds and fungus with vinegar. Spraying your feet helps prevent athletes' foot.
- Vinegar dissolves warts: Mix one part vinegar to one part glycerin into a lotion and apply daily to warts until they dissolve.
- Stubborn rings resulting from wet glasses being placed on wood furniture may be removed by rubbing with a mixture of equal parts of white distilled vinegar and olive oil. Rub with the grain and polish for the best results.
- Window washer: Simply wash with a mixture of equal parts of white distilled vinegar and warm water. Dry with a soft cloth. This solution will make your windows gleam and will not leave
- Brass, copper and pewter will shine if cleaned with the following mixture: Dissolve 1 teaspoon of salt in 1 cup of white distilled vinegar

and stir in flour until it becomes a paste. Apply paste to the metals and let it stand for about 15 minutes. Rinse with clean warm water and polish until dry.

- Bathtub film can be removed by wiping with white distilled vinegar and then with soda. Rinse clean with water.
- Rub down shower doors with a sponge soaked in white distilled vinegar to remove soap residue.
- To wash no-wax floors, add ½ cup of white distilled vinegar to a half-gallon of warm water.
- For spot less china or glasses: Pour 1½ cup to 2 cups white distilled vinegar in the bottom of dishwasher, along with regular dishwasher soap. Wash full cycle.
- Stubborn stains can be removed from the toilet by spraying them with white distilled vinegar and brushing vigorously. The bowl may be deodorized by adding 3 cups of white distilled vinegar. Allow it to remain for a half hour, then flush.
- In hard water areas, add a cup of vinegar to a gallon of tap water for watering acid loving plants like rhododendrons, gardenias or azaleas. The vinegar will release iron in the soil for the plants to use.
- Keep cut flowers fresh longer by adding 2 tablespoons sugar and 2 tablespoons white vinegar to a 1-quart vase of water. Trim stems and change water every five days.
- Remove bumper stickers by repeatedly wiping the sticker with white distilled vinegar until it is soaked. In a few minutes, it should peel off easily. Test on a small invisible area of the car to ensure there will be no damage to the paint.
- For those winter mornings when there is frost/ice on the car window, wipe the windows the night before with a solution of one part water to three parts white distilled vinegar. They won't frost over.
- If you have a worn DVD that has begun to stick or suffers from the occasional freeze-frame, wipe it down with white distilled vinegar applied to a soft cloth. Ensure the DVD is completely dry before reinserting in the DVD player. (Note: This only works on DVDs that are scratched or dirty through normal wear.)
- The addition of 1 cup of white distilled vinegar to each load of baby clothes during the rinse cycle will naturally break down uric acid and soapy residue leaving the clothes soft and fresh. This works for cotton and wool blankets and other fabrics too. Deodorant and antiperspirant

stains may be removed from clothing by lightly rubbing with white distilled vinegar and laundering as usual.

• For dandruff relief after shampooing, rinse with a solution of ½ cup vinegar and 2 cups of warm water.

• How to build a volcano: First, make the "cone" of the volcano. Mix 6 cups flour, 2 cups salt, 4 tablespoons cooking oil and 2 cups of water. The resulting mixture should be smooth and firm (more water may be added if needed). Stand a soda bottle in a baking pan and mold the dough around it into a volcano shape. Do not cover the hole or drop dough into it. Fill the bottle most of the way full with warm water and a bit of red food color (can be done before sculpting if you do not take so long that the water gets cold). Add 6 drops of detergent to the bottle contents. Add 2 tablespoons baking soda to the liquid. Slowly pour vinegar into the bottle. Watch out – eruption time!

If you want the best health possible remember, not for internal use!

OH NO, NOT BLACK PEPPER AND CONDIMENTS TOO?

"Reason, instead of being the ruler, has come to be the slave of appetite."* "It is impossible for you to increase in spiritual strength while your appetite and passions are not under perfect control."**

"In this fast age, the less exciting the food, the better. Condiments are injurious in their nature. Mustard, pepper, spices, pickles, and other things of a like character irritate the stomach and make the blood feverish and impure." White, E., Ministry of Healing, 1905:325.

How Does What You Eat Relate To Your Sanity?

Disordered eating in adolescents has been linked to suicidal thoughts. "Disordered eating" is a term that is used by some people to describe a wide variety of irregularities in eating behavior. Eating junk food, skipping meals or eating at irregular times are included in this definition. Poor eating habits and poor choices in the type of food eaten correlate with our brain chemistry, and thus, our very sanity.

It Cannot Be Scientifically Correct?

I've grown up being told of the dangers of black pepper. We never even had it our home as a child and still don't. I have seen people just pour black pepper on their food, even before they have tasted it. They have lost their un-perverted ability to enjoy wholesome foods. In my research for this article, 99% of the information available tells of black pepper's many benefits as a spice. Their defense is that it makes food more palatable, increases your appetite, stimulates the flow of digestive juices and has been used since the flood (thousands of years) without obvious injury, so it must be safe! So is it safe???

Black Pepper's History

Ground black peppercorn, usually referred to simply as "pepper" can be found on nearly every dinner table around the world, often alongside table salt. Pepper makes up 39% of all spice imports in the U.S. Salt is the number one spice import, at over 50%.

Along the spice trail to India, black pepper was like black gold. The ebony spice was so sought after in ancient times and in the Middle Ages that peppercorns could be substituted for currency and used to pay for everything from taxes to dowries. Black pepper's ability to spice up bland foods and disguise lack of freshness made it indispensable in the time before refrigeration and before the global spice trade made exotic seasonings common.

Black pepper is a perennial woody vine. Pepper comes from several species of a vinous plant, the spice being the fruit, called peppercorns. Black pepper is the dried, unripe berry. The corns are wrinkled and spherical, about 5 mm (1/8 in) in diameter. White pepper consists of the seed only, with the fruit removed. Green pepper is from the same fruit but is harvested before they mature.

The Negative Effects Of Black Pepper

Mustard, black pepper, horse-radish, cayenne and capsicum contain irritating non-volatile oils. Several studies report that black pepper causes an increase in parietal secretion of hydrochloric acid and pepsin and a loss of potassium in the stomach. Black pepper causes the acid to be produced in excess. Black pepper can produce heart burn, acid (sour) stomach, peptic ulcers, etc. Also, there are reports of mucosal micro-bleeding of the whole gastrointestinal tract (from mouth to exit) and gastric bleeding due to black pepper's effects.

"Spices at first irritate the tender coating of the stomach, but finally destroy the natural sensitiveness of this delicate membrane. The blood becomes fevered, the animal propensities are aroused, while the moral and intellectual powers are weakened, and become servants to the baser passions." White, E., Counsels on Health, 1890:114. How'd she know that?

Black pepper is eliminated from the diet of patients having abdominal surgery and ulcers because of its irritating effect upon the intestines, being replaced by what is referred to as a bland diet. It takes about a month to re-train your brain and taste buds. Yes, you can live without it.

The Dangers Of Piperine

The active ingredient in pepper is piperine.

1. Piperine is mildly carcinogenic by containing small amounts of safrole (also found in cinnamon and nutmeg). Safrole is banned as a food additive by the FDA. It is also banned for use in soaps and perfume by the FDA.
2. Piperine (containing safrole) is used as an effective insecticide.
3. Piperine might even have negative effects on sperm and interfere with reproductive processes.
4. Piperine has also been found to inhibit human CYP3A4. CYP3A4 is a member of the cytochrome P450 mixed-function oxidase system. CYP3A4 is found in the liver, intestine and brain. It plays an important role in the metabolism of toxins and certain drugs. Without it we will become toxic.
5. Piperine inhibits P-glycoprotein (human ABC-transporter/ATP-binding cassette sub-family B member-1). P-glycoprotein promotes the migration of dendritic nerve cells. So piperine can block the growth of nerve cells and thus slow or inhibit the body's electrical system. P-glycoprotein protects the hematopoietic (blood making) stem cells from toxins. Piperine can block your stem cells from working properly.

Eat Plain Wholesome Foods

"It is impossible for those who give the reins to appetite to attain to Christian perfection. The moral sensibilities of your children cannot be easily aroused, unless you are careful in the selection of their food. Many a mother sets a table that is a snare to her family. Flesh-meats, butter, cheese, rich pastry, spiced foods, and condiments are freely partaken of by both old and young. These things do their work in deranging the stomach, exciting the nerves, and enfeebling the intellect. The blood-making organs cannot convert such things into good blood. The grease cooked in the food renders it difficult of digestion. The effect of cheese is deleterious. Fine-flour bread does not impart to the system the nourishment that is to be found in unbolted wheat bread. Its common use will not keep the system in the best condition." White, E., Counsels on Health, 1890:114.

* White, E., Counsels on Diet and Foods,1890:149.
** White, E., Counsels on Diet and Foods,1870:63

References:
Mahoney, D., *"Disordered Eating Linked To Suicidal Thoughts,"* Internal Medicine News, July 1, 2008:30. http://en.wikipedia.org/wiki/Peppercorn_%28fruit%29
Clarke, Anne *"Black Pepper -- Benefits and Possible Risks."* Black Pepper -- Benefits and Possible Risks. 17 May. 2006.
EzineArticles.com. 5 Jul 2008 <http://ezinearticles.com/?Black-Pepper----Benefits-and-Possible-Risks&id=200086>.
Dean, Michael (2002-11-01). The Human ATP-Binding Cassette (ABC) Transporter Super family. National Library of Medicine (US), NCBI.
http://en.wikipedia.org/wiki/Piperine
http://en.wikipedia.org/wiki/Safrole
Safrole Toxcity: http://potency.lbl.gov/pdfs/herp.pdf

For further study: White, E., The Ministry Of Healing, "Diet and Health": 295310.

ICE CREAM
- Is It Poison?

My Dad used to say, "***You scream, I scream, we all scream for ice cream.***"*

The History Of Ice Cream

Before 1000 BC/BCE, the Chinese whipped together frozen cream, eggs and sugar to make the first recorded ice cream. It was introduced to Europe by Marco Polo. Legend has it that the Roman Emperor Nero (54-68 AD/CE) used to send slaves scurrying to the mountains to collect snow and ice to make flavored ices in the first century. The first written mention of ice cream in this country was in the 1700's when George Washington (who is said to have consumed enormous quantities) was a guest of the Maryland governor. The flavor was fresh strawberry. The first U.S. ice cream parlor opened in New York City in 1776. In 1846, New Jersey native Nancy Johnson invented the hand-cranked freezer. Americans consume the most ice cream in the world per capita, with Australians second. In 1924, the average American ate eight pints a year. In 1997, each American averaged 48 pints (8 gallons) a year.

Ice Cream Facts

Vanilla is the most popular flavor (20-29%), while chocolate comes in a distant second (9-10%). Immigrants at Ellis Island were served vanilla ice cream as part of their Welcome to America meal. One major ingredient in ice cream is air. Without it, the stuff would be as hard as a rock. One out of every five ice cream eaters share their treat with their pet (dog, cat and/or bird). Ice cream novelties such as ice cream on sticks and ice cream bars were introduced in the 1920's. Seems like kid's stuff, but today adults consume nearly half of all such treats.

Ice Cream Cone History

Italian immigrant, Italo Marchiony, is generally credited with first inventing the ice cream cone. As a New York City ice cream vendor, he created the cone in 1896 (some say September 22, 1886) to stop his customers from stealing his serving glasses. He patented the idea in 1903. Charles Robert and brother Frank Menches who ran ice cream concessions at fairs and events across the Midwest, also claimed to have invented the cone for the 1904 World's Fair in St. Louis. E.A. Hamwi, a Syrian immigrant pastry maker, also had a stand at the St Louis World's Fair and claimed to have invented the cone. He is said to have hit upon the idea when some neighboring ice cream vendors ran out of dishes for their treats. He rolled some of his wafers, called Zalabia, into cone shapes while they were still hot, then let them cool and sold them to the neighbors to use for serving ice cream.

The Ice Cream Story

In the old days ice cream was made of whole eggs, milk and sugar and then laboriously cranked out in the old home freezer. A serving of ice cream was only an occasional summer family treat. Today, you may be treating your family to poison. Unfortunately along with the ice, comes the refined sugar, highly refined wheat (maltodextrin) and a whole lot of scary chemicals. There are over 1400 flavorings, stabilizers, colors and emulsifiers used by commercial ice cream manufacturers. Ice cream manufacturers are not required by law to list the additives used in their products. Consequently, most ice creams are synthetic from start to finish, because it costs less to produce. Nearly all artificial food flavors and food colors come from coal tar! This is a substance from coal and petroleum. Coal tar is notorious as a causative agent in producing cancer of the stomach, bowel, kidney, liver, and other organs.

Vanilla Flavor

Category I is commercial vanilla flavoring made entirely of vanilla. Natural vanilla (which is pureed vanilla beans or vanilla bean extract) is much more expensive than artificial vanilla.

Category II (Vanilla flavored) is a combination of natural and artificial flavors.

Category III (Artificially flavored vanilla) is entirely artificial. Artificial vanilla flavoring is peperonal or vanillin. Peperonal is a chemical used to kill lice. Vanillin is made from the wastes of wood pulp and has no relationship to the vanilla bean.

Strawberry Flavor

Strawberry flavor is Benzyl Acetate, a synthetic chemical that tastes like strawberries. According to the Merck Index, an encyclopedia for chemists, this substance is extremely dangerous and can cause vomiting and diarrhea. It is a nitrate solvent.

Pineapple Flavor

Pineapple flavoring is Ethyl Acetate. It can cause liver, kidney, and heart damage. It is also used as a cleaner for leather and textiles. Its vapors have been known to cause chronic lung, liver, and heart damage.

Banana Flavor

Banana flavoring is Amyl Butyrate or Acrylic Acetate, which is also used as an oil paint solvent.

Cherry Flavor

Cherry flavoring is Aldehyde C17, an inflammable liquid which is used as aniline dyes, and in the manufacture of plastic and rubber.

Nut

Nut flavoring is Butraldehyde, which is one of the ingredients in rubber cement.

Stabilizers And Emulsifiers In Ice Cream

Stabilizers make ice cream smooth; and emulsifiers make it stiff, so it can retain air. Here are some of the chemicals used to stabilize and emulsify ice cream: Propylene glycol (also used in antifreeze), glycerin, sodium carboxyl methylcellulose, monoglycerides, diglycerides, disodium phosphates, tetrasodium pyrophosphate, polysorbate 80, and dioctyl sodium sulfosuccinate. Manufacturers use diethylene glycol instead of egg yolk; it is used in antifreeze and as a paint remover. Recent illnesses caused by diethylene glycol required the recall of foreign manufactured 4 oz tubes of tooth paste nation wide.

Oxidized Cholesterol – BAD

Stored foods that contain cholesterol (cholesterol only comes from animals, like eggs, cheese, milk or meat) can combine with oxygen in the air to form "Oxidized Cholesterol." Oxidation products, even in small amounts, can cause lethal damage to the cells that line your arteries in less than 24 hours, giving rise to hardening of the arteries, which can hasten heart attacks and strokes. Drs. Peng and Taylor, in Albany, New York found if as little as ½% of your blood cholesterol was oxidized, it would have a deadly effect on your blood vessels. They found the most harmful combination for oxidized cholesterol was sugar, milk and eggs. Next harmful was pancake mixes containing eggs, hydrogenated oils and dried powdered milk. The third most harmful was Parmesan cheese, follow by lard.

What Does Ellen White Say About Ice Cream?

"I frequently sit down to the tables of the brethren and sisters, and see that they use a great amount of milk and sugar. These clog the system, irritate the digestive organs and affect the brain." 1870, Testimonies to the Church, Vol. 2, 370.

"Especially harmful are the custards and puddings in which milk, eggs, and sugar are the chief ingredients. The free use of milk and sugar taken together should be avoided." 1890, Counsels on Health, 154. Ice cream is the most common form of custard in the U.S. today. How did she know that 100+ years ago?

* Popular song by Tom Stacks performed with Harry Reser's Six Jumping Jacks, recorded January 14, 1928.

References:

http://everything2.com/title/ice+cream Hay, J., *"Ice Cream-Lies,"* http://editor.nourishedmagazine.com.au/ articles/ice-cream-lies Baum, M.D., *"Origins Of Ice Cream Cone Are Lost In Folklore,"* CNN. com, Food News, September 22, 2000.

Davis, S.E., *"Thirteen Fun facts About Ice Cream,"* www.aol.drspock.com/article/0, 1510,5941+++,00.html Nedley, N., "Proof Positive," Ardmore, OK; 1999:72-75.

Peng, S.K., *"Effects On Membrane Function By Cholesterol Oxidation Derivatives In Cultured Aortic Smooth Muscle Cells,"* Artery, 1987;14 (2):85-99.

Hubbard, R.W., *"Atherogenic Effect Of Oxidized Products Of Cholesterol,"* Prog Food Nutr Sci 1989;13(1):17-44.

CANCER IN A CAN

"Countries with per capita annual consumption of more than 20 gallons of fizzy soft drinks, also had rising rates of esophageal cancer."
Kaplan, L., New Scientist, May 18, 2004.

The Soda-Pop Problem

But I don't drink that much, you say! Drinking the equivalent of a two liter soda per week works out to be approximately 26 gallons a year. Drinking a 20 ounce soda a day is approximately 57 gallons per year. I just had a good friend and colleague die of poorly differentiated adenocarcinoma of the esophagus and I wanted to know why! This may not be the cause of his cancer, but it makes a lot of sense to avoid sodas.

Soft Drink Overload

Since most cancers are linked to what we eat and drink, researchers began looking for major dietary changes over the last 50 years to find the cause for the rise in swallowing tube (esophageal) cancer. During that time, the volume of carbonated soft drinks drunk in the US has increased 450 percent. In 1946, the average soft drink consumption per person was 10.8 gallons. In 2000, that increased to 46.2 gallons per person. In the last 25 years, rates of swallowing tube adenocarcinoma have risen by 570 percent in white males (the group with the highest soda-pop consumption). The average American drinks more soda than water.

Soda Puts On The Pounds

In the Southern portion of the US, the average soda-pop consumption is 663 cans per year. If that is non-diet soda, there is about 1teaspoon per ounce of sugar per can; equaling about 62 pounds of sugar a year. Sugar filled drinks are one reason for frequent infections and colds. Sugar impairs the white cell's ability to fight infections. Not only is soda a health risk for cancer, but, the sweetener, high-fructose corn syrup, causes an increased danger of diabetes, heart disease, stroke, premature aging, inflammatory conditions and gout attacks. If you're drinking diet soda, studies showed that you ate more and gained more over time than the regular soda drinkers, because artificial sweeteners increased both hunger and appetite. Heavy consumption of carbonated beverages leads to obesity that leads to gastric reflux disease that leads to esophageal cancer. Obesity is associated with a statistically significant increase in the risk of GERD (Gastro-Esophageal Reflux Disease), erosive esophagitis and esophageal adenocarcinoma. The risk for esophageal adenocarcinoma is 2.1 times higher in persons with a Body Mass Index (BMI) of 25 or greater.* 12 ounces of soda contains 150 calories and can cause 30 pounds of weight gain per year. Not everyone is gaining that much weight, so they are cutting back on a well balanced diet and are actually malnourished.

Too Acidic

There is also a connection between soft drink consumption and bone loss, via the acidic soda leaching out the bone's alkaline bone reserves, causing their premature thinning and ultimate fracture at an earlier age.

What About The Caffeine?

Most soft drink addicts are hooked on the caffeine in the soda and will drink it continuously all day long. The most popular addict-promoting sodas are Mountain Dew, Pepsi, Coke and Dr. Pepper. I never see someone drinking root beer all day long, unless it is caffeinated. Watch the labels because now some root beers are caffeinated. Caffeine, in the form of tea, coffee, colas and even chocolate, is known to dilate the esophageal-gastric ring. This muscle ring holds the acidic stomach contents in the stomach after you swallow.

Your stomach has a protective lining against the digestive acid, but your esophagus does not. The caffeine dilatation then allows acidic contents back in the swallowing tube; causing a re-occurring burn-like injury each time you use this stimulant. Caffeine can cause headaches, indigestion, nervousness, irritability, sleeplessness and a rapid heart rate.

Mountain Dew Danger

Brominated oils are added to soft drinks. The bromide in "Mountain Dew" type products, including Orange Crush, Sun Drop and Fresca, competes with iodide for uptake and utilization by the thyroid gland, thus causing a thyroid deficiency (hypothyroidism). Many of my patients know that they are tired, have dry skin, are losing their hair, and are having trouble with their memory, but only think it is old age. In reality, they are low in active thyroid (T3). Bromide and bromine are plentiful in our environment, without drinking more in a soda. Brominated pesticides are sprayed on fruits and vegetables. Bromine containing drugs are used widely in asthma medications. Over the past 20 years, bromination of bakery products was implemented by food processors. Over the past 20 years, an increased prevalence of cancer of the thyroid and breast cancer has been observed in American women. Bromide toxicity, thyroid and breast cancer potential, are correlated to the tissue bromide levels. So don't drink Mountain Dew type products to add to your problems.

There Are Chemicals In My Drink?

Worldwide, people drink 20,600,00 tons of chemicals (color, flavor, preservatives) from soda-pop each year. That's nine pounds for every person in the world.

Esophageal pH 7 Vs. 4

Your esophagus pH should be close to your body pH-7.4. Studies have shown that drinking just one can of soda lowers the pH of your esophagus to less than 4.0 for 53 minutes. This itself should not cause you any harm, but two cans a day for over 20 years might; add the extra reflux caused by the caffeine and "we have a problem Houston." 57 gallons of soft drinks a year (an oversize 20 ounce bottle per day) would subject your esophagus to an additional 32,100 minutes of acid exposure a year.

Park Ridge Hospital tap water-pH 8.0

Decaf Starbucks Coffee-pH 4.0

Dark brown cola type drinks (Coke, Pepsi, Dr. Pepper, etc) - pH 2.4-2.8. These all have phosphoric acid in them.

Mountain Dew, Root Beer, Sierra Mist, Seven Up, Sunkist or like soda-pH 4.0

Are We Sure About This?

There is a steep rise in swallowing tube cancers in Westernized countries (US, Australia New Zealand, Western Europe and the United Kingdom), but the risk of esophageal cancer is unchanged in countries where fizzy drinks have not caught on, like Japan, India, Eastern Europe and China. "The surprisingly strong correlation demonstrates the impact of diet patterns on health trends," says Dr. Mohandas Mallath, head of the digestive diseases department at Tata Memorial Hospital, India. The effects took about 20 years to show themselves. This association cannot be taken as a casual link at this stage. More research is needed. There are a whole variety of things that occur in modern society that may cause this cancer besides soda. Having refrigerators in your home has been associated with cancer, but refrigerators don't cause cancer. Heavy consumption of carbonated beverages may be a marker for lifestyle or dietary choices that increase the risk of esophageal cancer!

How Is A Soda Dangerous?

Previous studies have shown that gastric reflux causes the esophagus to become acidic for long periods of time; but your esophagus should be alkaline. Gastric reflux is the most important factor for development of esophageal adenocarcinoma. If you drink 12 ounces of water, your stomach will distend 12 ounces. If you drink a fizzy carbonated drink, your stomach will distend to twice as much; maybe 24 ounces for an original 12 ounce soft drink. This distention causes reflux and the stomach contents are thrown back into your food pipe to burn and irritate it, often, but not always, causing heartburn. My friend who died of esophageal cancer had no symptoms, no heartburn, no reflux, until he found the cancer had spread to his liver. Over time this irritation causes the lining of the esophagus, in some people, to mutate into this cancer.

Watch Out For Mint

One last warning for those with diagnosed esophageal problems. Mint can dilate your esophageal-gastric muscle ring/sphincter and cause reflux of your stomach contents into your throat. Even mint tea. What do fine restaurants give you when you've finished your meal? Coffee and a mint or chocolate mint; which will relieve your feeling of being overstuffed by relaxing your esophageal sphincter, taking the pressure off of your full stomach.

The Tale Of Two Wolves - Galatians 5:16-26

One night an old Cherokee told his grandson about a battle that goes on inside of people. He said, "My son, the battle is between two wolves inside us all.

One is Evil. It is anger, envy, jealousy, sorrow, regret, greed, arrogance, self-pity, guilt, resentment, inferiority, lies, false pride, superiority and ego.

The other is Good. It is joy, peace, love, hope, serenity, humility, kindness, benevolence, empathy, generosity, truth, compassion and faith. The grandson thought about it for a minute and then asked his grandfather: "Which wolf wins?" The old Cherokee simply replied, "The one you feed."

* Your BMI is calculated by multiplying your weight (in pounds) by 705; divide this number by your height in inches; divide this number again, by your height in inches. BMI is not a good measurement for the very muscular, very young, pregnant or frail individual. A BMI greater than 25 is considered overweight, a BMI over 30 is considered obese.

References:

Digestive Disease Week Conference, New Orleans, May, 2004. Hampel, H., *"Meta-Analysis: Obesity And The Risk For Gastroesophageal Reflux Disease And Its Complications,"* Annals of Internal Medicine, 2005;143:199-211.

Mallath, M., Digestive Diseases Department, Tata Memorial Hospital, India; presenter

Bhattacharya, S., *"Drinking Soda Linked To Gullet Cancer Rise,"* New Scientist, 18, May, 2004.

Williams, D., *"Cancer In Can,"* Alternatives, August 2004; 105-106.

Vobecky, *"Effect of Enhanced Bromide Intake On The Concentration Ratio I/Br In The Rat Thyroid Gland,"* Biological Trace Element Research, 43:509-516;1994.

Eskandari, S., J Biol. Chem., 272:27230-8;1997.

Abraham, G., *"Iodine Supplement Markedly Increases Urinary Excretion Of Fluoride And Bromide,"* Townsend Letter, 238:108-9;2003.

Abraham, G., *"Orthoiodo supplementation: Iodine Sufficiency Of The Whole Human Body,"* Original Internist, 9:30-41;2002.

Butcher, D., *"Trouble In A Can (Or Bottle),"* The Tuning Fork, Arden SDA Church Health Letter, 2004.

RISK OF DEATH FROM MEAT

- You Are What The Animals Eat

As a health minded church we have advocated for over 150 years to become vegetarian, but many have ignored this counsel with deadly results! Few studies have evaluated long-term meat consumption or the relationship between meat consumption and the risk of cancer, heart attacks and stroke–until now!

The National Institute Health Study-March 2009

Men and women who eat higher amounts of red meat and processed meat have a higher risk of dying from cancer, heart disease, and stroke compared to those who eat less or none. Those who ate the most red meat took in about 4.5 ounces a day – the equivalent of a small steak and/or about 1.5 ounces a day of processed meats (about 2 slices of deli turkey). Cutting down on red meat and processed meat would result in a "meaningful saving of lives," says Barry Popkin, PhD. The non-vegetarian Dr. Popkin is The Carla Smith Chamblee Distinguished Professor of Global Nutrition at the University of North Carolina School of Public Health, Chapel Hill.

Who's Included?

500,000 men and women participated in the National Institutes of Health-AARP Diet and Health Study. Participants were between the ages of 50 and 71 when the study began in 1995, and all provided detailed information about their food intake. After 10 years, using the Social Security Administration's databases to track causes of death, 47,976 men and 23,276 women died.

So What's Considered Bad?

So what was included as bad: red meat included beef, pork, bacon, ham, hamburger, hot dogs, liver, pork sausage, steak, and meats in foods such as pizza, stews, and lasagna. White meat included turkey, fish, chicken, chicken mixtures, and other meats. Processed meat was either white or red meat that was cured, dried, or smoked; such as bacon, chicken sausage, lunch meats, and cold cuts.

Eating Red Meat Linked To Colon Cancer-2005

Colon cancer is the third most common cause of cancer in men and woman, killing 56,000 each year. This study included 148,610 adults aged 50 to 74 years, residing in 21 states with population-based cancer registries, who provided information on meat consumption in 1982 and again in 1992/1993 when enrolled in the Cancer Prevention Study II (CPS II) Nutrition Cohort. Follow-up from the time of enrollment in 1992/1993 through August 31, 2001, identified 1,667 incident colorectal cancers. Those who ate the most red meat and processed meats developed colon cancer; 30-40% more than those who did not.

Eating Red Meat Linked To Breast Cancer-2007

Post-menopausal women who had the highest intake of red meat, the equivalent to one portion a day (more than 57 grams), run a 56 percent greater risk of breast cancer than those who eat none. Women who eat the most processed meat, such as bacon, sausages, or ham, run a 64 percent greater risk of breast cancer than those who eat none.

Americans Will Eat Anything

But this information doesn't change one's habits. You and I will agree that we can't believe what people did eat on TV's Fear Factor. But even without the "unclean" foods (Lev 11) being eaten, Americans are consuming more "clean" meat than ever. In 2004 we ate over 221 pounds of meat and poultry per person, up from 199 pounds in 1990.Americans have come to expect low prices on their meat products and in order for the industry to turn a profit, most livestock are kept and slaughtered on factory farms, where animals are feed corn and soybean based feeds (10-30% of which is often radically different from what the animal would consume naturally). For example, feathers, poultry manure and waste bedding are all acceptable in cattle feed, according to the Food and Drug Administration; not to mention the added sanctioned "get big quick" hormones that are added to the feeds and passed on to the consuming public. Poultry may also be fed meat and bone meal ground down to an inexpensive, protein rich powder that encourages fast growth.

The Pathogens Are Killing Us

For the year 2005, there were 24 recalls of meat due to dangerous levels of pathogens, including listeria, E coli, and spinal column remains of a cow over 30 months old. We hear about E coli killing or permanently damaging people while eating at salad bars, but the E coli came from the meat being prepared on the same surface as the salad. But Hamburger Is OK?

Ground beef is often extracted by a process called "Advance Meat Recovery (AMR)," where carcasses are fed into a machine that strips soft tissue from the bone. Processed meats, such as pizza toppings and sausage are made this way. Consumer advocates warn that AMR increases the risk of spinal tissue (which can carry mad cow disease) could be included among the processed meats. The American Meat Institute counters that the cow spinal cords are removed from all carcasses before being stripped.

Meanwhile, the first case of mad-cow disease in domestic-raised beef was discovered in Texas, June 2005.

Meat Is A Bacteria Magnet

Ground beef is the worst bacteria magnet. During the grinding process and packaging, it's exposed to air that is rife with harmful bugs including listeria, staphylococcus and salmonella. It is so difficult to prevent infection that the USDA says ground beef with 7.5% incidence of salmonella bacteria vs. 1% for raw cuts of meat.

Where'd My Meat Come From?

After Canada confirmed cases of mad cow disease in 2003, consumers wanted to know the country of origin of their meat products. Despite having a USDA stamp on the meat it still could have come from Argentina, Australia, Canada, Brazil or Mexico. These countries often do not meet the core requirements of the US law. The USDA's zero tolerance policy for contaminants including feces and urine were repeatedly violated by Australia, Canada and Mexico, the consumer watch-dog group Public Citizen warned in 2003. There is no country of origin label on meat. Unclean Stores

According to the New York Department of Agriculture, 25.5% of the state's department supermarkets were cited in 2004 for a critical deficiency involving insect, rodent, bird or vermin activity that had contaminated the meats. 7.5% were cited for unsanitary equipment services. Another 1% of the stores were cited for employees not washing their hands. We may need to start to have bathroom police here at church for not washing your hands and proceeding out to shake hands!

But, What About The Protein?

Alright, I hear some of you say, but what about the protein that our bodies need? Studies have for years suggested that meat eaters had higher blood pressure than vegetarians. A recent study (January 9, 2006) found that hypertension may partially be due to the type of protein we eat. Eating vegetable sources for your protein lowered your blood pressure. This was found to be true in 17 diverse populations and four countries. Eating a meat based diet or a high protein type diet did not over a long period change one's blood pressure, despite what the weight loss books say. In vegetable based protein diets, it is the different amino acids in the vegetable vs. meat proteins and increases in potassium and magnesium in the vegetable based diet, that cause the lowering of the blood pressure.

Meat Makes Us Spiritual Weaklings

"Flesh was never the best food; but its use is now doubly objectionable,

since disease in animals is so rapidly increasing." 1905,Counsels On Diet And Foods: 384

"Subsisting on the flesh of dead animals is a gross way of living..." 1884, Counsels On Diet And Foods: 409

"The Lord would bring His people into a position where they will not touch or taste the flesh of dead animals. Then let not these things be prescribed by any physicians who have a knowledge of the truth for this time." 1898, Counsels On Diet And Foods: 409.

"The unhealthful food placed in the stomach strengthens the appetites that war against the soul, developing the lower propensities. A diet of flesh meat tends to develop animalism. A development of animalism lessens spirituality, rendering the mind incapable of understanding truth." 1902, Counsels On Diet And Foods:382

References:

Sinha, R., *"Eating Red Meat Boosts Death Risk,"* Archives of Internal Medicine, March 23, 2009.

Thun, M, *"Red Meat Linked To Colon Cancer,"* JAMA, January 11, 2005; Vol 293, No.2: 172-182.

(Breast Cancer) http://www.sciencedaily.com/ releases/2006/11/061113180252.htm

Black, J, *"10 Things Your Butcher Won't Tell You,"* Smart Money, November 2005:110-112.

Elliot, P. *"Association Between Protein Intake And Blood Pressure,"* Arch Intern Med, 166; Jan. 9, 2006;79-87. White, E., "Counsels On Diet And Food," 1938.

THE URGE TO EAT

Why Am I So Hungry?

Americans have a love affair with food. Usually fried or sugary is most craved. At a recent first grade anti-obesity class in Henderson County, NC, over half of the pupils ate fast food daily. Many were unaware that this might be unhealthy. Also, some children had been told by their parents not to drink water because it was unhealthy, so they drank soda instead. Many obese children and adults are ravenously hungry all the time. Nothing the family or doctors say or do can keep them from constantly eating and therefore, from getting fatter.

Survival Of The Fattest

The miracle every one is looking for is something that makes fat melt off our bodies. Such is the dream of very dieter: a treatment that makes you slim by magically suppressing your hunger. Why do some people get fat and why do others stay thin? People who efficiently store food in the form of fat were the ones most likely to survive famines and pass on their "thrifty" genes (like the bedouins in the Middle East today).Those that stored their food for lean times didn't need to store their food as fat, and their genes reflected that. So some people genetically really can eat all they want and stay thin. They may be the genetic oddity, though. Most of us have a genetic profile that leads us to get fat when there's plenty of food.

Is Obesity Glandular Or Hormonal?

Popular diets have fostered the myth that obesity is due to the lack of willpower. Our genetic profile plays a big role in determining how fat we are, as it does determining our ultimate height. Fat cells communicate with the brain (saying more chocolate, more French fries) via a hormone found in 1994, called leptin. Leptin is part of a complex system that regulates body fat and hunger. When we put on fat, fat cells release leptin, which signals the brain to suppress your appetite. When we burn fat, leptin levels fall, and the hunger center of the brain (thalamus) says," eat something."

Resistant To The Hunger-Suppressing Hormone-Leptin

There are a few obese people (exceedingly rare) that genetically lack the ability to make leptin, and when supplied with leptin they dramatically lose weight. Scientists thought they had found the dieters magic bullet. Paradoxically, 90% of obese people actually have high levels of leptin and are resistant (the brain is not responding to the leptin). Some scientists have even suggested that leptin's trouble reaching the brain is from fat particles (triglycerides) gumming up the blood-brain barrier, making it hard for leptin to get across. Triglyceride levels rise as people gain weight, thus preventing leptin from reaching the brain, they say. The lack of leptin makes people feel that they are starving and they eat more, adding even more fat, which increases their leptin resistance and makes them hungrier.

Causes For Weight Loss Failure

There are other factors besides leptin that cause people to become overweight, but resistance to this hormone makes losing weight very hard.

'Resistance to leptin' people need more leptin to suppress their appetites. But as fat cells shrink, the bodies' leptin levels fall and that triggers hunger pangs and slows the metabolism. The brain responses as if one were in a famine, conserving energy and ordering you to eat, eat, eat. Thus, shedding pounds and keeping them off can be very difficult. This is why so many people that lose weight will gain it right back. Low and high metabolisms run in families. Many overweight people can survive on 500 to 1000 calories a day by this leptin-fat cell mechanism.

Appetite's Two Opposites: Ghrelin/Stimulant vs. PYY/Suppression

Ghrelin is produced in the stomach and is a hunger hormone. As we diet and lose weight, ghrelin levels increase. Ghrelin is one of the reasons we regain that weight after we have lost it. Ghrelin's opposite hormone is Peptide YY3-36 (PYY), a hormone produced in the intestines, which promotes satiety (being full). When PYY is low in humans, they are more likely to be overweight. PYY (appetite suppression) infusions produced a fall in ghrelin (appetite stimulant) and thus weight loss. Ghrelin levels fall after gastric bypass surgery, because the stomach is "bypassed." Researchers are hoping to market a pill that has leptin and PYY in it for post weight loss/dieters to be able to keep off the pounds.

The Fat Causing Virus

In 2002, an analysis of 1000 people with antibodies (a sign of being infected) to the human adeno-virus-36 (AD-36) were significantly more likely to be overweight. AD-36 is a "cold" virus. AD-36 injected into monkeys caused dramatic weight gain. In some animals the virus caused their weight to triple. So can a virus make you fat? When fat cells are exposed to AD-36 they begin to multiply. Obesity is caused by your genes, metabolism and habits, and now add infection. A vaccine has been suggested, if AD-36 antibodies are found to be widespread. Now, another reason to wash your hands regularly to prevent this cold virus!

Fidgeters Lose Weight

Your weight depends on how much you eat and how much you move. Researchers have found another trait that determines how fast we burn calories: fidgeting. Some people tap their fingers or jiggle their legs more than others. This tendency runs in families. Natural fidgeters are more sensitive to calories. They unconsciously increase their activity level after they eat too much and tended to weight less than those family members who did not fidget and ate the same amount of food.

Our Choice

We can't pick our parents or change our genes, but we can change our environment. It is up to us what we eat and don't eat. It is up to us if we watch an hour of TV or go for a walk. But hunger cues via our hormones are so strong that even the steeliest will power isn't enough to resist eating, in many people. So here are some tips:

- Pray without ceasing
- Exercise decreases your appetite.
- Increasing your water intake decreases your appetite.
- Increasing your fiber intake decreases your appetite.
- Eating very little or raw veggies for your evening meal resets your hunger drive.
- During stressful times eat more protein, not calorie rich fats and sugars.

Unready For The Loud Cry

"The health reform, I was shown, is a part of the third angel's message, and is just as closely connected with it as are the arm and hand with the human body." White, E.G., "Unready For The Loud Cry," Testimonies To the Church, Vol.1; 1867:486-487.

"Gluttony is the prevailing sin of this age. Lustful appetite makes slaves of men and women, and beclouds their intellects and stupefies their moral sensibilities to such a degree that the sacred, elevated truths of God's word are not appreciated. The lower propensities have ruled men and woman. In order to be fitted for translation, the people of God... should ever have the appetite in subjection to the moral and intellectual organs. The body should be servant to the mind, and not the mind to the body." White, E.G., "Unready For The Loud Cry," Testimonies To the Church, Vol.1; 1867:486-487.

"Whatever may be our inherited (genetic, in your DNA) or cultivated (habits, brain circuitry, reprogramming your DNA) tendencies to wrong, we can overcome through the power that He is ready to impart." White, E.G., Ministry Of Healing, 1905:176.

DO YOU BELIEVE THAT!?

References:

Jaret, P., *"Beating The Urge To Eat,"* Readers Digest, rd.com; July2004:118-123

Atkinson, R.L, *"Human Adeno-virus-36 Is Associated With Increased Body Weight And Paradoxical Reduction Of Serum Lipids,"* International Journal of Obesity, 2005;29:281-286.

Joyal, S., *"Leptin, Ghrelin And PYY3-36: Magic Bullets Or Blanks?"* physicalmag.com, Feb 2003:52-55.

Lemonick, M., *"Lean And Hungrier,"* Time; June 3,2002:54.

FIGHTING DISEASE WITH YOUR FORK

- Permanent Healthy Weight Loss
- The Garden Of Eden Raw Food Diet
- Live Food, Live Body; Dead Food, Dead Body

You've tried all the latest fad diets. You're worried about getting the Big C (cancer). You need to reduce your grocery bill. What are you going to do?

An Early Death From The Great American Diet

3rd world countries don't have the diseases that we have on the 'Great American' diet of high sugar and low fiber, processed and fried foods. 3rd world countries eat a diet rich in natural/raw foods. They don't get breast, colon and prostate cancers. They don't have heart burn, hiatal hernias, peptic ulcer disease, gallbladder disease, diverticulosis, constipation, hemorrhoids, or varicose veins. They rarely have heart attacks and strokes. Why? Because they eat a high fiber (raw), low-sugar, alkaline diet. You've heard me say if you become too acidic you will die. Staying alkaline is the key to health and the best way is through a raw food diet.

You Want Me To Eat What?

It may be hard to believe, but most people in the United States are over weight and most people in the United States are suffering from malnutrition. I don't recommend diets, because they fail. I recommend life style change. A 50% raw food diet is an easy way to start that change in your life. Wow, that's a lot of raw food, but the successful "Hallelujah Acres Raw Food Diet" is 85% raw and 15% cooked food. Hallelujah Acres is like Weimar (a health retreat), without the spiritual component. With my Crohn's disease I have found that I always do well with raw celery and raw carrots. Both are hypo-allergic.

So What Can I Eat On A Raw Diet?

Fresh fruits (limit fruit to 15% of daily food intake), vegetables, raw nuts, raw and sprouted seeds, beans, soaked grains, sprouted legumes, dried fruit (unsulphured), seaweed, olives, avocados, olive and flaxseed oils, fresh and dehydrated herbs, garlic, sweet onions, parsley and salt free seasonings, unprocessed organic or natural foods, freshly juiced fruit and vegetables, and purified re-mineralized water. Dairy alternatives include: almond/rice/soy milk, creamy banana milk, frozen fruit (banana, strawberry, blueberry, etc) creams, tahini, non-dairy cheeses and soups made from scratch without fat, dairy or additives you cannot pronounce.

Why Is A Raw Food Diet Better Than What I'm Eating Now?

God has given us an abundance of natural healing foods, unprocessed and uncooked plants, such as fresh fruit and vegetables, sprouts, seeds, nuts, grains, beans, nuts, dried fruit, and seaweed. There is a major Ph (acid/base) shift in your physiology with raw foods which makes you feel highly energized. A large part of cooked food can only go into fat production, because heat and acid alter it, making it un-metabolizable in other complex processes. By contrast, raw food breaks down into components which can be directly metabolized into a variety of our cells. These dense living nutrients found in raw foods and their juices are what meet and satisfy our cells' nutritional needs. The benefits of a raw food diet include: increased energy, improved skin appearance, better digestion, natural weight loss and a reduced risk of heart disease and stroke. A person on this 'diet' no longer needs to struggle with uncontrollable hunger. These live foods are what produce abundant energy and vibrant health.

Lose Weight With A Raw Food Diet

Health advocates have suggested that we need to eat more fiber for years. It scrubs your bowels of toxins, decreases the risk of diverticulosis and of colon cancer. It lowers your cholesterol by binding to the cholesterol and preventing it from being absorbed. You burn 7 calories for every gram of fiber you eat. At 35 grams per day (recommended amount of fiber/day), you'll neutralize 250 calories per day. That's 15 pounds you'll lose per year without changing any other of your routines.

Less Heart Disease, Diabetes And Cancer In A Raw Food Diet

The raw food diet contains no trans fats, no cholesterol and less saturated fat than the typical Western diet. It is also low in sodium and high in potassium, magnesium, folate, fiber and health-promoting plant chemicals called phytochemicals. These properties are associated with a reduced risk of diseases such as heart disease, diabetes, and cancer. For example, a study published in the Journal of Nutrition found that consumption of a raw food diet lowered plasma total cholesterol and triglyceride concentrations.

Elevated Homocysteine And Low B12 Levels Do Not Come From This Diet!

Some scientists have suggested that a raw food diet will cause B12 deficiency and an elevated homocysteine level. Very little B12 is needed in this type of diet and B12 is produced by the microbes in our intestines. Our microbes change depending on what we eat. So the right diet will have the right B12 producing microbes. I never have seen an elevated homocysteine level in a person who eats plenty of green veggies which are a rich source of folic acid; folic acid lowers homocysteine levels.

Getting Started

There are thousands of exciting recipes on the internet. Start your healthy new year with a raw food treat.

References:

Koebnick C, Garcia AL, Dagnelie PC, Strassner C, Lindemans J, Katz N, Leitzmann C, Hoffmann I. *"Long-term consumption of a raw food dietis associated with favorable serum LDL cholesterol and triglycerides but also with elevated plasma homocysteine and low serum HDL cholesterol in humans,"* J Nutr. 2005 Oct;135(10):2372-8.

Hallelujah Diet: HYPERLINK "http://www.hacres.com" www.hacres.com

www.Rawfoods.com

DO YOU WANT CANCER WITH THOSE FRIES?

- Three Cancer Studies Reviewed

Weight Gain Can Correlate With Breast Cancer

A woman's weight gain after age 18 correlates with her risk of breast cancer. Woman who gained 30 to 40 pounds between the ages of 18 and 57 were 40% more likely to get breast cancer than woman who gained five pounds or less. Women who gained more than 70 pounds had twice the risk. Fat cells make their own estrogen, so heavier people have higher estrogen levels. Higher estrogen increases breast cancer risk.

French Fries And Breast Cancer

The Nurses Health Study found that women were more likely to get breast cancer if they had regularly eaten French fries decades earlier as preschoolers. This is a long term health study of 25,000 nurses. In this particular arm of the study, 582 nurses who had breast cancer in 1993 were compared with 1569 nurses who didn't have breast cancer. Their mothers were asked how often the nurses had eaten 30 different foods as preschoolers. French fries were the only food associated with a higher risk of breast cancer. Foods not linked in this study with breast cancer include cheese, butter, ground beef and cookies. For every extra weekly serving of French fries that the women reportedly ate as preschoolers, their risk of breast cancer as adults rose 27 percent.

Did These Moms Really Remember What Their Children Ate 40 Years Ago?

Problems with this study could be people's memories. Moms in their 60's, 70's and 80's remembering what their children ate decades ago surprises me. These moms did know that their daughters had breast cancer when being interviewed, so did that change their answers?

Saturated Fats And Trans Fats As Cause?

This study spans over 40 years and there has been a wide range of French fry making during that time. Some woman may have eaten fries baked at home in lard (rich in cholesterol and saturated fats). Others may have eaten fast food French fries cooked in oils high in trans fats. Cancer can take decades to develop. Breast tissue (both male and female) prior to puberty is much more susceptible to environmental and potentially cancer causing influences than adult breast tissue. Men account for 1% of all breast cancer.

Back To The Garden Of Eden Diet

Physicians are already concerned about children's diets and the rising epidemic of childhood obesity. Here is one more reason to watch a child's diet, so that when they grow up they do not suffer from a variety of chronic diseases.

Acrylamide Danger

Cancer causing chemicals are found in most of our food sources. Acrylamide is an industrial chemical used in plastics, pesticides and sewage treatment that can occur when starchy foods are processed at high temperatures. Acrylamide is formed during preparation of bread, coffee, breakfast cereals, chips and other fried, baked or roasted high-carbohydrate foods. Raw food materials used in these foods have shown no trace of acrylamide. Eating foods fried at high temperatures or for along time should be avoid.

Potato Chip Risk

An ordinary bag of potato chips may contain up 500 times more acrylamide than the top level allowed in drinking water by the World Health Organization (WHO). That means that eating a single potato chip may contain enough acrylamide to equal the maximum allowed for drinking water. Research has shown that most chip manufacturers have unsafe levels of acrylamide in their products. A study looked at one ounce servings, which ranged from 11 to 20 chips depending on the brand, and determined the acrylamide content was substantially more than the daily acceptable level.

French Fry Risk

French fries sold at Swedish franchises of U.S. fast food chains Burger King and McDonald's contained 100 times the one microgram per liter of acrylamide maximum permitted by WHO (2002). The Environmental Protection Agency (EPA) wants this chemical listed on these products that are to be consumed. WHO has said acrylamide maybe responsible for up to one-third of all cancers caused by our diet.

Probable Human Carcinogen

Acrylamide is currently classified as a probable human carcinogen because, in high doses, it has been found to induce gene mutations that can cause benign and malignant stomach tumors in laboratory animals. It is also known to cause damage to the central and peripheral nervous system. Acrylamide is on California's list of chemicals known to cause cancer and required by Proposition 65, in that state, to be listed on packaged products.

What To Do?

Processed foods are known to contain carcinogens caused by heat processing. So what are we to do? Go back to the Garden of Eden type diet. Avoid processed, high carbohydrate, deep fried foods.

References:

Feigelson, H.S., *"American Cancer Society"* reported in Cancer Epidemiology, Biomarkers & Prevention, 2004.

Michels, K., *"French Fries In Childhood Tied To Breast Cancer?"* International Journal of Cancer, online edition, March 29, 2006.

Starck P., *"Cancer Risk Found In French Fries, Bread,"* www.reuters.com, April 24, 2002 From Stockholm University with Sweden's National Food Administration.

WHY DO I KEEP GAINING WEIGHT?

You exercise and watch what you eat but you are still gaining weight-why? Your metabolism rate is the largest factor in determining your weight loss success. What slows metabolism down? As you age, your muscle mass decreases and therefore, so does your metabolic rate.

Your Metabolism Slows By 5% Every Decade

Your metabolic rate is made up of three parts: 70% is your Basal (resting) Metabolic Rate (BMR), 10% is the thermal effects of the food you eat and 20-25% is made up by your physical activity. "If you never had problems losing or maintaining your weight in your 20s or even in your early 30s, you may not be ready for what happens next," warns Madelyn H. Fernstrom, Ph.D., director of the Weight Management Center at the University of Pittsburgh Medical Center. "Your metabolism slows by 5 percent each decade. Compared to age 25, you'll burn about 100 fewer calories a day at 35 and 200 fewer at 45. Do nothing and you could gain eight to 12 pounds a year." One pound of fat burns 2 calories per day at rest, while a pound of muscle burns 6-12 calories during the same period. When you add exercise, your muscles burn a lot more calories, while your fat continues to burn two calories per pound no matter what you do.

Muscle Burns Three Times More Calories Than Fat

"A woman who weighs 130 pounds and has a healthy 25 percent body fat will burn about 200 more calories per day than a 130-pound woman with about 40 percent body fat — a typical level for women at mid life," says David C. Nieman, Dr., P.H., director of the Human Performance Laboratory at Appalachian State University in Boone, NC. You can go to a local gym or your fitness center to be measured for your body percentage of fat. Anything over 30% fat needs attention.

How Many Calories Can I Eat Without Gaining Weight?

It takes energy to maintain your bodily functions like digestion, blood circulation, and breathing. The energy, or calories, you burn just to keep you alive is called your BMR. It mirrors how many calories you would burn if you did nothing all day but lie in bed. So here's the formula to calculate your BMR:

- Women: 655 + (4.35 x weight in pounds) + (4.7 x height in inches) - (4.7 x age in years)
- Men: 66 + (6.23 x weight in pounds) + (12.7 x height in inches) - (6.8x age in years)

OK, so how many calories do I burn if I am:

- Sedentary (little or no exercise): BMR x 1.2
- Lightly active (easy exercise/sports 1-3 days/week): BMR x 1.375
- Moderately active (moderate exercise/sports 3-5 days/week): BMR x 1.55
- Very active (hard exercise/sports 6-7 days a week): BMR x 1.725
- Extremely active (very hard exercise/sports and physical job): BMR x 1.9

This is the total number of calories per day you would need to eat to maintain your current weight. If this sounds too easy, it is. It depends on the percentage of lean body muscle and body fat that you start with!

One pound of body fat is equivalent to 3,500 calories — which means a person must cut that many calories from their diet to lose a single pound of fat. Eliminate 500 calories a day by reducing your calorie intake by 300 calories a day and increase your activity to burn 200 extra calories per day and you can expect a steady weight loss of approximately one pound per week. Here are the most common mistakes affecting your metabolic rate.

Mistake #1: Crash Dieting

A fast can drop your metabolic rate by as much as 25 percent. If you're on a very-low-cal diet (400- to 800-calories a day) your metabolic rate falls by 15 to 20 percent. Eating fewer than 900 calories a day burns desirable muscle tissue as well as fat, which slows your metabolic rate even more. If your diet stays within the 1,200 to 1,500 calorie range, about 90 percent of the weight you lose will be fat and you'll lower your metabolic rate only by about 5 percent.

Amino Acid Leucine

Eat about 20% of your diet as protein. Protein contains leucine, one of the eight essential amino acid, that protects you from muscle loss during dieting. Foods rich in leucine include: soybeans, seeds, peanuts, almonds, walnuts, chickpeas, garbanzos, flax seed, hummus and asparagus.

Mistake #2: Never Challenging Your Muscles

If you never exercise you will lose up to five pounds of muscle each decade. You need to exercise - walking, biking, swimming, or sweating at an exercise class. Strength training causes micro-tears in your muscles and rebuilding them burns a lot of calories and fat. After ten weeks strength training 20 minutes twice a week, women showed an added 2.6 pounds of muscle and lost 4.6 pounds of body fat.

Mistake #3: Never Changing Your Routine

Researchers at the University of Guelph in Ontario found that women who did interval workouts on stationary bikes for two weeks burned 36 percent more fat than when they completed a steady ride. Martin Gibala, Ph.D., and exercise physiologist at McMaster University says, "When you push hard in short bursts, it reactivates nerve fibers, builds new capillaries, and forces your body to repair the muscle. All of that burns a tremendous amount of calories," for up to eight hours afterwards.

Mistake #4: Being Sleep Deprived

When Harvard Medical School scientists followed 68,183 women for 16 years, they found that those averaging five hours of sleep a night were 32 percent more likely to gain 33 pounds than those who got seven hours a night. Those sleeping an average of six hours per night were 12 percent more likely to gain weight. Sleep deprivation increases the appetite-stimulating hormone, ghrelin, and decreases the satisfaction hormone, leptin, say researchers from the University of Chicago. In a study they conducted, tired volunteers craved more candy, cookies, chips, and pasta.

Mistake #5: Being Stressed Out

When you get hurried and stressed (Job! Kids! House! Marriage!), your levels of cortisol (a stress hormone), go up. That triggers cravings for high-fat, high-carbohydrate foods and sends that extra fat to your (Oh, NO!) waistline. All that extra cortisol makes you want to eat–anything and everything. Avoid starchy food in the last half of the day. Choose low glycemic index carbs for your carbohydrate portions. If you will take a walk, look at greenery, drink water, call a friend, read, or pray, the 'urge to splurge' will pass in 10 to 20 minutes.

Drink your allotment of water. ½ your weight in pounds = ounces per day of water intake you should drink. Not only will this decrease your appetite, but it will lessen your stress level. Add 16 ounces of water for very cup of tea, coffee, or soda you drink. So I recommend you avoid these beverages and stick to water to stay hydrated and decrease your perceived stress level.

Mistake #6: Forgetting To Eat Breakfast

You overate at supper, so you have no appetite in the morning. So you're trying to cut calories early in the day; but women whose diet resolve is strongest in the morning reset their metabolism lower to burn 5% less calories by skipping breakfast. Missed meals decrease the receptors in your brain and stomach that register satisfaction and fullness. Researchers at the University of Texas at El Paso discovered a metabolic appetite control: a hearty breakfast. Study volunteers who ate a bigger meal in the morning went on to eat 100 to 200 fewer calories later in the day. Research from Michigan State University that tracked 4,218 people showed that women who skipped breakfast were 30 percent more likely to be overweight. So eat healthy and have a good breakfast!

Rejoice evermore. Pray without ceasing. In every thing give thanks: for this is the will of God in Christ Jesus concerning you.
1Thesssalonians 5:16-18

References:

Harrar, S., *"Supercharge Your Metabolism,"* April 2008:173-174; 250.http://www.goodhousekeeping.com/health/advice/boost-metabolism-lose-weight

Provost, J., *"How Many Calories Do You Need?"* April 2008 www. goodhousekeeping.com/bmr

http://www.weightlossforall.com/calories-per-pound.htm

http://www.personaltrainingfitness.com/calories-per-pound-of-fat.html

OBESITY AND MSG

- Is There A Trigger In Our Diet?
- Excitotoxins And High Fructose Corn Syrup

Additives

Food processing tactics are changing constantly. New chemical additives are being introduced to improve shelf life, enhance color, enhance flavor and improve the mouth feel (texture), all the time. It staggers the mind that these different additives, preservatives, artificial colors, flavors and sweeteners might interact with our bodies to cause us harm.

MSG Triples Insulin Release

Does MSG (Monosodium Glutamate) really cause a tripling of the production of insulin the pancreas makes? The FDA has declared MSG safe in any amount. But the answer is, YES! Too much insulin causes you to eat more so you don't get hypoglycemia (low blood sugar). My patients with hypoglycemia consume larger amounts of refined carbohydrates than they normally would, to counteract the overproduction of simulated insulin. The more insulin you produce in your life time, the harder it is on your body, and researchers report it causes you to age quicker.

MSG's In Everything?

MSG is in most processed foods, either labeled as MSG or as one of these ingredients: autolyzed yeast, calcium or sodium caseinate, gelatin, hydrolyzed protein, yeast extract, textured protein, carrageenan, vegetable gum, seasonings, spices, flavorings, natural flavorings, chicken flavoring, beef flavoring, bouillon, pork flavoring, smoke flavoring, broth, stock, barley malt, malt extract, malt flavoring, whey protein, whey protein isolate, soy protein, whey protein concentrate, soy sauce, soy protein isolate, soy protein concentrate and soy extract.

Why Add MSG?

MSG is always present in any gelatin-encapsulated vitamin or supplement. It is in soups, chips/Doritos, Top Ramen, boxed helpers/ mixes, gravy, frozen dinners, and salad dressings (especially the low fat ones). It is used at Burger King, McDonalds, Wendy's, Taco Bell, TGIF, Chilis', Applebee's, KFC and Denny's. Why is MSG added to our foods? To make us eat more. The MSG manufacturers themselves admit that it addicts people to their products. It is like nicotine in our food. It makes people chose their product over another and eat more of their product than if it didn't have MSG in it. Thus, MSG causes obesity and it is addictive! MSG is being added in larger and larger doses to prepackaged meals, soups, snacks and fast foods to make us eat more.

MSG Is Addictive

Monosodium glutamate is a neurotransmitter. Glutamate is a highly regulated chemical of the nervous system, and a proper balance is necessary for healthy brain and organ function. In fact, every major human organ is now known to contain glutamate receptors.

Over stimulation of these receptors—in the brain or elsewhere—can lead to numerous health problems, many of which may mimic other disorders (such as fibromyalgia or heart arrhythmia), but can go undiagnosed for decades; all the while creating a life of misery and disability for the hypersensitive sufferer.

Are You Excitotoxin Sensitive?

Many of us may be suffering needlessly because of so-called "safe" food additives, namely excitatory neuro-transmitters (nicknamed excitotoxins). The main ones are monosodium glutamate (MSG), aspartame, and L-cysteine. They can contribute to a positive review of your body systems and include: headaches, migraines, stomach upset, nausea and vomiting, diarrhea, irritable bowel syndrome, asthma attacks, shortness of breath, heart palpitations, partial paralysis, mental confusion, anxiety or panic attacks, balance difficulties, neurological disorders (mimics Parkinson's, MS, ALS, Alzheimer's), heart attack-like symptoms, behavioral disorders (especially in children and teens), allergy-type symptoms, skin rashes, mood swings, runny nose, bags under the eyes, flushing, mouth lesions and depression.

Artificial Sweeteners

If you're drinking or eating diet (sugar free) drinks or foods, studies have shown that you will eat more and gain more weight over time; when all the time we thought it would help us lose weight! The reason is because artificial sweeteners increase both your hunger and your appetite. Sweeteners that cause you to still be hungry after eating are: saccharin (Sweet and Low®; pink packs), aspartame (Nutrasweet® and Equal®; blue packs), Stevia Extract (green packs), and Splenda® (yellow packs). New artificial sweeteners are introduced every few years and are quickly blended into everything from soft drinks to pancake mix. So, if you want to lose some weight, read the labels, and avoid these substitute sweeteners!

High Fructose Corn Syrup (HFCS)

In 1996, HFCS was introduced into our foods. A sudden increase in obesity and diabetes has been seen since then, worldwide. HFCS causes an increased danger of heart disease, stroke, premature aging, inflammatory conditions and gouty attacks. HFCS is the number one sweetener in the U.S., with sales of over $4.5 billion dollars a year. The average American consumes 62 pounds of HFCS a year (year 2002). HFCS is also found in ketchup, relish, cookies, jelly, syrups, baked goods, fruits and desserts.

Leptin And Ghrelin

Your body processes HFCS much differently than it does plain beet or cane sugar. When sugar is ingested, the pancreas releases insulin, which helps move the sugar from the blood stream into cells. The insulin also causes fat cells to release the compound leptin, which results in the feeling of "fullness" and, at the same time, prevents the release of a compound from the stomach called ghrelin, which makes a person feel hungry. Fructose doesn't trigger the release of leptin from fat cells, or suppress the release of ghrelin. Therefore, with HFCS products you may never feel satisfied or full, and you may stay hungry despite consuming a large amount of calories. One can see how this could cause an increase in caloric intake and ultimately unwanted weight gain. Put another way, consuming foods and drinks with HFCS increases your hunger, causes you to eat more than you normally would, which in turn causes you to gain weight.

HFCS Increases Your Changes of Diabetes

HFCS does not have a first pass liver blood sugar rise, like table sugar. HFCS, more so than glucose, is converted by the liver into triglycerides. High triglycerides levels tend to increase levels of LDL cholesterol (bad), lower levels of HDL cholesterol (good), and block insulin receptors. Persistent high triglyceride levels correlate with insulin resistance, a procurer of diabetes.

Irritable Bowel Syndrome (IBS) And HFCS

10-20% of the US suffers from IBS. IBS is defined by having a non pathological cause of bowel complaints which include:

- abnormal stool formation-alternating hard or loose stool,
- abnormal frequency-either more than three per day or fewer than three per week,
- abnormal stool passage-straining, extreme urgency, or the feeling of not being able to completely evacuate,
- passage of mucous,
- bloating or the feeling of being bloated.

Dr. Choi Young, of the University of Iowa Carver College of Medicine, tested 183 people over two years. He consistently found that each of the symptoms of IBS could be triggered with an increased use of HFCS and would disappear by avoiding HFCS. He felt that 30-60% of all cases of IBS are related to HFCS.

A Work Of A Life Time

"All our habits, tastes, and inclinations must be educated in harmony with the laws of life and health. By this means we may secure the very best physical conditions, and have mental clearness to discern between the evil and the good." White, E., "The Christian Race," Counsels on Diet and Foods, 1890:28.

References:

Williams, D., *"When Good Guts Go Bad,"* October 2005;11(4):25-32.
Young, C., Gastroenterology, 2003;98(6):1348-1353.
www.truthinlabeling.org (MSG and artificial sweeteners)
www.nomsg.com
www.msgmyth.com
Erb J., *"The Slow Poisoning Of America"* www.spofamerica.com.

SUGAR:
YOUR IMMUNE SYSTEM AND HEART DISEASE

- Don't Blind Your White Cells
- Your Diet, Mood, Stress and Genetics All Play A Role

"Most people worry that they eat too much between Thanksgiving and Christmas, when really they should be worried about eating too much between Christmas and Thanksgiving." Anonymous

The chance of dying from cancer, heart disease, stroke, viral or bacterial infections, like pneumonia, depend on the strength of your immune system. We could all die, if it were not for our immune system's ability to fight foreign invaders and chronic inflammation in our body. Our immune system's response depends on our diet, stress, genetics and our mood. Our nutrition can up regulate or down regulate our genes for life or death.

We have a raw cooking school starting January 11 here. Every Sunday from 3-5pm. Don't miss it.

Getting A Cold Or The Flu?

Around the holidays people tend to eat more sugary foods and refined carbohydrates, thus, having a direct and negative effect on their immune system. Adults tend to get 2-4 colds or flu a year. The common cold's increased occurrence is when the air is colder and less humid, we don't get as much sunshine (vitamin D) and is more common around the holidays when our defenses are down from our intemperance in our diet.

Holiday Cheer Or Holiday Fear

Increased sugar intake boosts the neurotransmitter serotonin, our happy mood brain chemical. This suggests that eating sugar can make you feel better when you are depressed. Your mood may temporally improve from the sugar high; but, you will pay a high price. Numerous research studies have shown that increased sugar intake dramatically decreases your immune response. Short-term hyperglycemia (high blood sugar) negatively affects all major components of your immunity.

Sugar Blinds Your Immune System

Your white cells (leukocytes) are the primary mediators of the immune response. Neutrophils are a type of white blood cell that is a first line of defense that swallows up (phagocytosis) foreign cells or bugs. High sugar loads in the body turn off the neutrophils radar for several hours, depending on the amount of sugar ingested. High glucose levels increase the risk of infections from Staphylococcus epidermidis, Staphylococcus aureus and E coli. In diabetics, high glucose levels increase the risk of Klebsiella pneumoniae. In healthy adults, eating simple carbohydrates like: glucose, fructose, sucrose, honey and orange juice significantly decreased the ability of the neutrophil to engulf bacteria. The greatest effect was one to two hours after the sugar consumption, but lasted for up to five hours before the fasting control values of normal white cell function returned to normal.

Sugar And Heart Disease

But sugar doesn't cause heart disease? Can it? The Atherosclerosis Risk in Communities Study (ARIC), a community-based cohort of almost 16,000 people from four states (North Carolina, Mississippi, Maryland and Minnesota), found that HbA1c levels taken in 1990-1992 and tracked for 10-12 years, correlated with coronary heart disease events, hospitalizations and deaths.

HbA1c Predicts Heart Disease

Hemoglobin A1c (HbA1c) is a measure of the amount of sugar attached to your hemoglobin molecule and thus, a measure of your long-term blood glucose level. Researchers found that HbA1c predicts heart disease risk in both diabetics and non-diabetics. An elevated blood glucose level is the defining feature of diabetes. It has been argued whether elevated glucose levels contributed independently to increasing heart-disease risk, until now! In participants with diabetes, the researchers found a graded association between HbA1c and increasing coronary heart disease risk. Each 1-percentage-point increase in HbA1c level was associated with a 14 percent increase in heart disease risk. Non-diabetic persons with HbA1c levels of 6 percent or higher had almost a two-fold greater heart disease risk compared to persons with an HbA1c level below 4.6 percent.

Stress And Your Immune System

Stress, through the hypothalamic-pituitary-adrenal axis, modulates the immune system. The adrenal glands produce cortisol in response to stress, which suppresses the immune response. Stress can reduce neutrophil activity, change the type of chemical mediators called cytokines produced by the white cells, decrease cytotoxic T-lymphocytes (CD8) and natural killer cells. It is now known that increased stress can lead to increased respiratory infections, due to a stress related decrease in your immune response.

What Can I Do? Seven Recommendations

Recommendation #1: Cut out the sugars and refined carbohydrates in your diet and eat more raw food to improve your immune system function.

Vitamin A is required for the growth and activation of B-lymphocytes, increases macrophages, improves T-lymphocyte function and is critical in maintaining sufficient levels of natural killer cells.

Recommendation #2--5,000 IU of Vitamin A a day extra while sick. Vitamin C can reduce the duration and frequency of the viral common cold and flu symptoms.

Recommendation #3--1000 mg of Vitamin C every several hours, no maximum.

Vitamin B6 improves lymphocyte differentiation, maturation and antibody production.

Recommendation #4--100 mg of B6 a day, maximum.

Zinc improves white cells immune function such as neutrophils, natural killer cells, T lymphocyte function and B lymphocyte development, antibody production and macrophage activity.

Recommendation #5–add an extra 15 mg of zinc a day. Literature suggests that greater than 100 mg a day of zinc actually depresses the immune system.

Vitamin D up-regulates the gene called cathelicidin, a naturally occurring broad spectrum antibiotic in our white cells.

Recommendation #6--5000 IU of Vitamin D a day.

Recommendation #7--Read your Bible daily for its healing qualities.

Recommendation #8 *"A merry heart doeth good like a medicine, but a broken spirit drieth up the bones."* Prov 17:22

References:

Zabriskie, N., *"Holiday Immune Support: Sugar+Stress = Vulnerability To Colds And Flu,"* Vitamin Research News,, Nov 2008;22(11):1-5.

Reiche, E.M., *"Stress And Depression-induced Immune Dysfunction: Implications For The Development And Progression Of Cancer,"* Int. Rev. Psychiatry, Dec 2005;17(6):5150527.

Selvin, E., *"Meta-Analysis: Glycosylated Hemoglobin and Cardiovascular Disease in Diabetes Mellitus,"* Archives of Internal Medicine, September 12, 2005;14(6):421-431.

Smolders, I., *"Effects Of Dietary Sucrose On Hippocampal Serotonin Release,"* Britsh J Nutr., August 2001;86(2):151-5

Patel, K.L., *"Impact Of Tight Glucose Control On Postoperative Infection Rates And Wound Healing In Cardiac Surgery Patients,"* J Wound Ostomy Continenced Nurs., Jul-Aug 2008;35(4):397-404.

Alba-Lourerio, T.C., *"Neutrophil Function and Metabolism In Individuals With Diabetes Mellitus,"* Braz J Med Biol Res, Aug 2007;40(8):1037-44.

Rall, L.C., *"Vitamin B6 And Immune Competence,"* Nutr Rev, Aug 1993;51(8):217-25.

Gorton, H.C., *"The Effectiveness Of Vitamin C In Preventing And Relieving The Symptoms Of Virus-induced Respiratory Infections,"* J Manipulative Physiol Ther., Oct 1999; 22(8):530-3.

Mossad, S.B., *"Zinc Gluconate Lozenges For Treating The Common Cold: A Randomized, Double-blind, Placebo-controlled Study,"* Ann Intern Med., Jul 1996;125(2):81-8.

Cannell, J.J., *"Epidemic Influenza and Vitamin D,"* Epidemiol Infect., Dec 2006; 134(6):1129-40.

Cannell, J.J., *"Use Of Vitmain D In Clinical Practice,"* Altern Med Rev., Mar 2008;13(1):6-20.

Recent Health Nuggets at ParkRidgeCardiology.com

SUGAR SUBSTITUTES

Are artificial sweeteners safe? The succession of new artificial sweeteners has claimed at first to be healthy, only later proven to be full of side effects. As food additives, artificial sweeteners are not subject to the same gauntlet of FDA safety trials as pharmaceutical medications. Most of the testing is funded by the food industry, which has a vested interest in the outcome. People have been using artificial sweeteners for decades. Studies show that people who use artificial sweeteners in place of sugar eat more calories and gain more weight because these sweeteners increased both their hunger and appetite by blocking their brain's satiety center. Some people react poorly to sweeteners, some don't. The problem is you may never know until you're already sick! Artificial sweeteners are body toxins. They are never a good idea for pregnant women, children or teenagers, despite the reduced sugar content, because of possible irreversible cell damage.

Artificial Sweeteners

Saccharin: (Sweet and Low®-pink packet) In 1879, Ira Remsen,a researcher from Johns Hopkins University in Baltimore, Md., noticed that a derivative of coal tar he accidentally spilled on his hand tasted sweet. Saccharin is a protoplasmic poison. No matter how long it takes, saccharin eventually kills protoplasm. It has induced bladder cancer in mice and rats, and produced deformities in developing chicks. Saccharin kills amoeba (one celled animals), in one part to 8000 parts water, in less than 24 hours. Saccharin 1:10,000 is approximately the mix one gets when you add one 'pink' package to your cup of coffee or tea.

Aspartame: (Nutrasweet®, Equal®-blue packet and its cousin, Neotame, FDA approved July 9, 2002) has been known to cause obesity, menstrual problems, brains lesions, and possible tumors. People who are sensitive to processed free glutamic acid (MSG) experience similar reactions to aspartame. One of our doctor's wives quit using this product and it markedly improved her daily headaches. Aspartame triggers the body's conversion of blood glucose into saturated fats (which increase your cholesterol numbers), thus causing low sugar. European research shows that ingesting aspartame leads to the accumulation of formaldehyde in the brain, other organs and tissues. Formaldehyde has been shown to damage the nervous system, immune system, and cause irreversible genetic damage in humans.

One out of 20,000 babies is born without the ability to metabolize phenylalanine, one of the two amino acids in aspartame. This can cause mental retardation.

It can worsen seizures, depression and Parkinsonism by phenylalanine competing with levadopa for uptake into the human brain. If you use Sinemet (carbidopa/levadopa), Stalevo, Parcopa, or a like product, don't use aspartame.

When heated (as little as 86° F) or left open to air, it breaks down into toxic chemicals including wood alcohol (methanol), which can cause blindness. Aspartame is not to be used in cooking.

Splenda: (sucralose-yellow packet) is 600 times sweeter than table sugar and is used in over 15% of all foods and beverages sold in the US. Splenda is the trade name for sucralose, a synthetic compound stumbled upon in 1976 by scientists in Britain seeking a new pesticide formulation.

It is true that the Splenda molecule is comprised of sucrose (sugar) except that three of the hydroxyl groups in the molecule have been replaced by three chlorine atoms.

The manufacturer of Splenda claims that the chlorine added to sucralose is similar to the chlorine atom in the salt (NaCl) molecule. Chlorine is nature's Doberman attack dog, a highly excitable, ferocious atomic element employed as a bio-cide in bleach, disinfectants, insecticide, WWI poison gas and hydrochloric acid. However, sucralose may be more like ingesting tiny amounts of chlorinated pesticides; but we will never know without long-term, independent human research. Experts say Splenda has more in common with DDT than with food. Reported side effects of Splenda include: skin rashes/flushing, panic-like agitation, dizziness and numbness, diarrhea, muscle aches, headaches, intestinal cramping, bladder issues, and stomach pain.

Acesulfame potassium (acesulfame K or Ace-K; Sold as Sunett, Sweet n' Safe or Sweet One) was discovered in 1967, but has only been FDA available since 1988. It is a calorie-free sweetener that is 200 times sweeter than sugar. It is not metabolized or stored in the body. The organic intermediate, Acetoacetic acid, when combined with the naturally occurring mineral, potassium, forms this highly stable (can be heated), crystalline sweetener.

Acetoacetic acid in concentrations of 1-5% in the diet of rats for several months caused thyroid tumors, which raises serious questions about its carcinogenic potential. Acesulfame stimulates insulin secretion in a dose dependent fashion thereby possibly aggravating reactive hypoglycemia ("low blood sugar attacks"). Acesulfame K apparently produced lung tumors, breast tumors, rare types of tumors of other organs (such as the thymus gland), several forms of leukemia and chronic respiratory disease in several rodent studies, even when less than maximum doses were given; yet was approved for human consumption.

Natural Sweeteners

Gaio® D-Tagatose: (Sold as Gaio Sugaree) D-Tagatose was produced by inventor Gilbert V. Levin in 1967, by Spherix. He is also famous for his work with NASA on the 1976 Viking Mars Lander. "It looks like sugar, tastes like sugar, cooks like sugar," because this sugar is not from cane or sugar beets but from a dairy by-product: whey. Unlike ordinary sugar, it has no calories. Nor will it decay teeth. It strengthens beneficial bacteria in the gastrointestinal track. You can bake with it and use it to caramelize. It is slightly less sweet than table sugar. D-Tagatose is a ketohexose sugar, with a similar structure to fructose, and is naturally present in small amounts in heat-treated dairy products, like yogurt, and found in soy products and even human breast milk. It has the potential to induce glycogen deposits and hypertrophy of the liver and to increase the concentrations of uric acid in your blood serum, which can cause gout. When consumed in large amounts, people experience gastrointestinal distress, including diarrhea, nausea and flatulence, because it is not digested or absorbed.

Fructosamine: better known as corn syrup, does not produce a first pass liver blood sugar rise. It becomes glyceride, which can increase your triglycerides. High triglycerides block insulin receptors. This causes high insulin blood levels, which makes you insulin resistant, thus leading to full blown diabetes. So, high-fructose corn syrup can cause an increased danger of diabetes, heart disease, stroke, premature aging, inflammatory conditions and gout attacks. It is twice as sweet as sugar and can be used in cooking.

Agave Syrup: is no better than refined sugar. Agave is being used in more of our foods and beverages. It has 20 calories per teaspoon compared to only 16 calories per teaspoon of table sugar. It contains up to 90% fructose, depending on the way it is processed. Agave has more fructose than in high-fructose corn syrup. Even though it is marketed as 'diabetic friendly,' there are no studies to support this claim. Some studies have suggested that large amounts of fructose can increase the risk of diabetes and can have harmful effects on the heart and liver.

Polyalcohol Sugars

These include: **Sorbitol, Xylitol, Malitol,** and **Mannitol**. These are natural sweeteners that do not trigger an insulin reaction. They have half the calories of sugar, taste like sugar and are not digested by the small intestine. Sorbitol is a natural laxative and can cause diarrhea, irritable bowel syndrome, bloating and flatulence. Xylitol comes from birch tree pulp and corncobs. It also reduces tooth plaque and helps build tooth enamel.

My Choice For You

Lo Han Kuo: (Siraitia grosvenori) may be sold as Lo Han Sweet. It is an extract from a dried fruit that has been cultivated since the 13th century in Southern China. It is 300 times sweeter than sugar and has no calories. Lo Han Kuo helps to control food and sugar cravings, helps digestive tract problems, sore throats, chronic coughs, constipation, headache, and tension. It is being marketed to compete with Stevia, but is hard to find. It can be purchased from the internet through the distributor Jarrow.

Stevia: (Stevia Rebaudiana-green packet or liquid) was discovered in 1887 by scientist Antonia Bertoni via the Guarani Paraguayan Indians, who have used it for over 400 year. Stevia is from a small native plant/ herb in Paraguay and Brazil. Stevia is extracted from the leaves to a substance 300 times sweeter than table sugar. It has almost no calories, can be used in baking, is non toxic, but does have an herb-like after-taste. For a sugar substitute, it is my choice for my patients.

THE TOP 10 FOODS THAT FIGHT FAT

- Fiber Fights Fat Eat More Fiber

For years, health scientists have suggested that we need to eat more fiber. It scrubs your bowels of toxins, decreases the risk of diverticulosis. It lowers your cholesterol by binding to the cholesterol and preventing it from being absorbed. Did you know that you burn 7 calories for every gram of fiber you eat? At 40 grams per day (recommended amount of fiber/day), you'll neutralize 250 calories per day. That's 15 pounds you'll lose per year without changing any other of your routines. The average American eats 3-10 grams of fiber a day. So eat more fiber, drink more water*, and stop eating when you are no longer hungry. It is advocated that you eat nine (9) pieces/serving of fruit or vegetable every day. This will easily get you past the 40 gram a day of fiber we all need. Now, if you add 10 more minutes of exercise (like walking), you will lose weight with this simple plan.

*drink one ounce of water for every kilogram (pounds/2.2) of your body weight each day.

THE POWER OF APPETITE

- The Dangers Of Meat Eating -By Ellen G. White

"One of the strongest temptations that man has to meet is upon the point of appetite. Between the mind and the body there is a mysterious and wonderful relation. They react upon each other. To keep the body in a healthy condition to develop its strength, that every part of the living machinery may act harmoniously, should be the first study of our life. To neglect the body is to neglect the mind. It cannot be to the glory of

God for His children to have sickly bodies or dwarfed minds. To indulge the taste at the expense of health is a wicked abuse of the senses. Those who engage in any species of intemperance, either in eating or drinking, waste their physical energies and weaken moral power. They will feel the retribution which follows the transgression of physical law." Counsels on Health 122.1

Teach The Little Ones

"Self-denial should be taught to children and enforced upon them, so far as is consistent, from babyhood. Teach the little ones that they should eat to live, not live to eat; that appetite must be held in abeyance to the will; and that the will must be governed by calm, intelligent reason." Counsels on Health 113.1

Meat Develops Animalism In Man

"The unhealthful food placed in the stomach strengthens the appetites that war against the soul, developing the lower propensities. A diet of flesh meat tends to develop animalism. A development of animalism lessens spirituality, rendering the mind incapable of understanding truth." Counsels on Health 575.4

God's Original Plan

"It is not the chief end of man to gratify his appetite. There are physical wants to be supplied; but because of this is it necessary that man shall be controlled by appetite? Will the people who are seeking to become holy, pure, refined, that they may be introduced into the society of heavenly angels, continue to take the life of God's creatures, and enjoy their flesh as a luxury? From what the Lord has shown me, this order of things will be changed, and God's peculiar people will exercise temperance in all things." Counsels on Health 116.2 *"Again and again I have been shown that God is trying to lead us back, step by step, to His original design--that man should subsist upon the natural products of the earth. Among those who are waiting for the coming of the Lord, meat eating will eventually be done away; flesh will cease to form a part of their diet. We should ever keep this end in view, and endeavor to work steadily toward it. . . ."* Counsels on Health 450.1

Disease Increased Ten Fold By Eating Meat

"The liability to take disease is increased tenfold by meat eating. The intellectual, the moral, and the physical powers are depreciated by the habitual use of flesh meats. Meat eating deranges the system, beclouds the intellect, and blunts the moral sensibilities. . . . Your safest course is to let meat alone."--Testimonies for the Church, vol. 2, pp. 63, 64 (1868).

Evils Of Meat Eating

"Those who use flesh meats freely do not always have an unclouded brain and an active intellect, because the use of the flesh of animals tends to cause a grossness of body and to benumb the finer sensibilities of the mind. The liability to disease is increased by flesh eating. We do not hesitate to say that meat is not essential to the maintenance of health and strength." Counsels on Health 115.1

Diseased Meat

"Those who subsist largely upon meat cannot avoid sometimes eating flesh which is more or less diseased. In many cases the process of fitting animals for market produces an unhealthy condition. Shut away from light and pure air, inhaling the atmosphere of filthy stables, the entire body soon becomes contaminated with foul matter; and when such flesh is received into the human body it corrupts the blood, and disease is produced. If the person already has impure blood, this unhealthful condition will be greatly aggravated. But few can be made to believe that it is the meat they have eaten which has poisoned their blood and caused their suffering. Many die of diseases wholly due to meat eating, when the real cause is scarcely suspected by themselves or others. Some do not immediately feel its effects, but this is no evidence that it does not hurt them. It may be doing its work surely upon the system, yet for the time being the victim may realize nothing of it." Counsels on Health 115.2

The Danger Of Pork

"Pork, although one of the most common articles of diet, is one of the most injurious. God did not prohibit the Hebrew from eating swine's flesh merely to show His authority, but because it is not a proper article of food for man. God never created the swine to be eaten under any circumstances. It is impossible for the flesh of any living creature to be healthful when filth is its natural element, and when it feeds upon every detestable thing." Counsels on Health 116.1

Higher And Lower Nature Affected

"The unhealthful food placed in the stomach strengthens the appetites that war against the soul, developing the lower propensities. A diet of flesh meat tends to develop animalism. A development of animalism lessens spirituality, rendering the mind incapable of understanding truth. The word of God plainly warns us that unless we abstain from fleshly lusts, the physical nature will be brought into conflict with the spiritual nature. Lustful eating wars against health and peace. Thus a warfare is instituted between the higher and the lower attributes of the man. The lower

propensities, strong and active, oppress the soul. The highest interests of the being are imperiled by the indulgence of appetites unsanctioned by Heaven." Counsels on Health 576.1

The Temptation Of Meat

"Satan tempted them (Israel in the Old Testament) to regard this restriction as unjust and cruel. He caused them to lust after forbidden things, because he saw that the unrestrained indulgence of appetite would tend to produce sensuality, and by this means the people could be more easily brought under his control. The author of disease and misery will assail men where he can have the greatest success. Through temptations addressed to the appetite he has, to a large extent, led men into sin from the time when he induced Eve to eat of the forbidden fruit. It was by this same means that he led Israel to murmur against God. Intemperance in eating and drinking, leading as it does to the indulgence of the lower passions, prepares the way for men to disregard all moral obligations. When assailed by temptation, they have little power of resistance." Patriarchs and Prophets 378

Feverish Influence Of Meat

"Meat should not be placed before our children. Its influence is to excite and strengthen the lower passions and has a tendency to deaden the moral powers. Grains and fruits prepared free from grease, and in as natural a condition as possible, should be the food for the tables of all who claim to be preparing for translation to heaven. The less feverish the diet, the more easily can the passions be controlled. Gratification of taste should not be consulted irrespective of physical, intellectual, or moral health." Counsels on Health 621.2

Criminal Behavior From Diet

"Indulgence of the baser passions will lead very many to shut their eyes to the light, for they fear that they will see sins which they are unwilling to forsake. All may see if they will. If they choose darkness rather than light, their criminality will be none the less. Why do not men and women read, and become intelligent upon these things, which so decidedly affect their physical, intellectual, and moral strength? God has given you a habitation to care for and preserve in the best condition for His service and glory. Your bodies are not your own. "What? know ye not that your body is the temple of the Holy Ghost which is in you, which ye have of God, and ye are not your own? For ye are bought with a price: therefore glorify God in your body, and in your spirit, which are God's." 1 Corinthians 6:19, 20. *"Know ye not that ye are the temple of God, and that the Spirit*

of God dwelleth in you? If any man defile the temple of God, him shall God destroy; for the temple of God is holy, which temple ye are." 1 Corinthians 3:16, 17." Counsels on Health 622.1

Our Witness

"We are not to make the use of flesh food a test of fellowship, but we should consider the influence that professed believers who use flesh foods have over others." Counsels on Health 133.3

References:

White, E.G., Counsels on Health, Complication of Health Principles written over 40 years (1868-1909), Pacific Press Publishing Association, 1951.

White, E.G., Patriarchs and Prophets, Pacific Press Publishing Association, 1958.

White, E.G., Testimonies for the Church, Vol. 2, Pacific Press Publishing Association, 1948 Edited by Royce Bailey MD

OMEGA-3 FATTY ACIDS

Why So Much Fuss About Omega's

Essential Fatty Acids (EFAs) serve as building blocks of nerve cells and cell membranes. Without friendly fats, dangerous saturated fats will replace EFAs in the cell's membrane coat. This can cause reduced membrane fluidity and efficiency. This then is the start of premature aging and disease development.

Eicosapentaenoic Acid (EPA)
Docosahexaenoic Acid (DHA)

EPA/DHA blood levels (less than 1.2% vs. greater than 2.6% of total fatty acids) correlated with the cardio-protective effect of Omega-3s. The recommended Omega-3s to achieve high blood levels is 1400 mg EPA and 1000 mg DHA.

DHA is derived from marine sources and algae or a break down of alpha linolenic acid-ALA to the active EPA/DHA.

Omega-3 Has Anti-Inflammatory Effects

Thousands of studies are clear that we don't get enough Omega-3 in our diet. Its benefits include a strong anti-inflammatory effect that inhibits prostaglandin E2 (PE2). PE2 contributes to blood vessel inflammation, and as been implicated in the formation of vulnerable arterial plaques that may rupture and cause death. Other anti-inflammatory processes which may be helped include: arthritis, cancer,

Crohn's disease, diabetes, Alzheimer's disease, peripheral neuropathy, psoriasis, cardiac dysrrhythmias (atrial and ventricular), PMS and depression, to name a few.

Eat freshly ground flax seed two tablespoons full each day. Don't grind a couple of days worth at once; because the oil is so unstable it will be rancid in a couple of hours if not readily consumed, even if kept in the refrigerator. Omega-3 are also found in walnuts, pecans and raw seeds, but there is not much Omega-3 in almonds.

Breast Cancer

Breast cancer incidence in laboratory rats decreased by 30% when supplemented with DHA. DHA supplements increased the BRCA1 protein produced by a major tumor suppressor gene by 60%. Omega-3 activates a gene that confers breast cancer protection. This supports the literature observation that high Omega-3 intake may reduce the risk of breast cancer.

Mood And Brain Volume

Higher intake of omega-3 fatty acids is associated with greater volume in areas of the brain related to mood and behavior. Magnetic Resonance Imaging (MRI) were used to measure gray matter volume in the brains of 55 adults. Subjects with higher Omega-3 intake had greater gray matter volume in areas of their brains associated with emotional arousal and regulation. These same areas were reduced in volume in people with mood disorders, such as major depressive disorders.

Danger Of Flaxseed Oil

Flaxseed, a source of Omega-3 fatty acids (alpha linolenic acid-ALA) and lignan, has been shown to inhibit melanoma, breast cancer, and prostate cancer growth. Two tablespoons of freshly ground flaxseed a day decreased free testosterone and cholesterol levels by day 2143. Low grade prostate disease had a decreased cell proliferation in the flaxseed groups, but a recent study of 47,000 men showed that flaxseed oil may worsen advanced prostate cancer. The reason was high levels of ALA did not convert to the beneficial EPA/DHA Omega-3. EPA (eicosapentaenoic acid) and DHA (docosahexaenoic acid) are polyunsaturated fatty acids that are part of the Omega-3 family and are found in cold water fish. The enzyme delta six desaturase converts ALA to EPA/DHA, but delta six desaturase is severely inhibited by elevated insulin levels. Thus, anyone with diabetes type 2 that is over weight with high cholesterol or high blood pressure can have elevated insulin levels and should not take flax seed oil for their cancer!

References:
Jourdan, ML, *"Increased BRCA1 Protein In Mammary Tumours Of Rats Fed Marine Omega-3 Fatty Acids,"* Oncol Rep, Apr 2007;17(4):713-9.
www.upmc.com/communications.NewsBureau/
NewsRelaeseArchives/2007/March/Omega3
improvesmood.htm. Am J Clin Nutr, July 2004;80(1):204-216.

THIS LITTLE PIGGY . . .

"And the swine, though he divide the hoof, and be cloven footed, yet he cheweth not the cud; he is unclean to you." Leviticus 11:7

"There Are No Absolutes," Satan Says

Satan's deceptions through the ages have flip-flopped. In the Dark Ages he pictured God as a tyrant, unmerciful, giving out punishment to all but a hand full of undeserving people. The Law of God was to be followed at all cost (justice), with no knowledge of a personal Savior. Now, Satan portrays God as too kind to harm anyone (mercy). I have had people tell me that "God would never destroy me. He's going to save everybody. So it doesn't matter what I do or eat. "There are no absolutes in this existential life," they tell me.

Acts 10 And 11

- Peter Instructed There Is No Difference Between Clean (Jews) and Unclean (Gentiles)

"You can eat what ever you want, because the Bible says so in the New Testament," I am told. This is the thinking I see when those that want no responsibility interpret Acts 10 and 11; because God in a vision to Peter reportable meant you could eat anything now (clean or unclean). These same folks say it's OK, because this vision freed us from the Law. Those laws were for the Jews. Interpretations like this contradict the Bible and scientific logic. Acts 10 and 11 have nothing to do with food!!!

"The great sin of the Jews was their rejection of Christ; the great sin of the Christian world would be their rejection of the Law of God, the foundation of His government in heaven and earth." White, E.G, "Great Controversy," Pacific Press Pub Ass., 1911:22.

The Pork Tapeworm-Taenia Solium

April 2001-Mayo Clinic in Scottsdale, AZ, doctors surgically removed a dead worm (cysticercosis-the pork tapeworm) from the brain of a woman. The greatest problems from this worm come from infections of the brain and eyes. The problem in treating "Taenia solium," is drugs kill the worm, which then releases all of its eggs. The doctor must then deal with the problem the eggs cause too. This lady had eaten infected pork while in Mexico. The worm had entered her brain and died. Its carcass was causing her periodic seizures (causing a foreign body reaction-like a piece of glass in your skin). The operation to remove the worm took six hours. It required that the patient be only mildly sedated, because she needed to be able to keep talking to surgeons to help guide them from point to point in her brain.

Trichinosis-Trichinella Spiralis

A patient of mine developed aching and inflammatory muscle pains, and later was diagnosed by me as having trichinosis. She became disabled at the age of 50, because of the encapsulated larva that had become embedded in her muscles from eating pork over the years. She is now a vegetarian, the only treatment that mildly helps the pain, she says. If she eats poorly (junk food and sweets) the pain will increase. She states, "If only I had started life as a vegetarian, like you."

Muscle Pain

My father, a surgeon, told me of the time an Orthodox Rabbi had come for an evaluation of his aching muscles and fevers, and that no one had been able to find the cause. My father biopsied a muscle on his arm and had him come back to the office for the results. He asked him in front of his wife if he ever ate pork. "Oh, no I would never do that, it's against the Torah!" Later, out of hearing of his wife, he said," Oh, Doc, please don't tell my wife, but I just love pork and eat it almost daily." He now had his diagnosis and was told that treatment of long-term cases was poor.

The Truth About Pork

My father had found from the biopsy that this Jewish man had trichinosis. 90% of trichinosis in the U.S. comes from eating pork and 10 % from eating bear meat. The larvae enter skeletal muscle where it grows between muscle fibers and begins to cause pain in several days. The severity of the infection depends on the number of larvae in the muscles (tens of thousands). By 6 to 18 months the cysts are calcified and therefore can cause severe pain with movement of the muscles. I am sure that many a patient has been mis-diagnosis as having fibromyalgia, when they really have trichinosis.

Does God Mean What He Says?

Is God arbitrary? Can justice and mercy be seen in our Savior at one time? Does He really want what is best for His people-Jewish or not? Should God's principles (like in Leviticus 11) be done away with? Ask someone with trichinosis!

References:
Shepard, C., *"News Of The Weird,"* www.mountain.com.; May 23-26, 2001:18.
Harrison's Textbook Of Medicine, 9th ed, McGraw-Hill,1980; *"Trichinosis," "Cysticercosis"*:894-5, 915-6.

PINE NUTS AND WEIGHT LOSS

The fatty acid pinolenic acid, found in pine nuts, can initiate the release of two appetite-suppressing hormones called "cholecystokinin (CCK)" and glucagon-like peptide (GLP-1), researchers have said. These two hormones send "satiety signals" to your brain that the stomach is full. CCK was increased by 65%, and GLP-1 was increased by 25% in those studied. Women in the study reported a lower desire to eat and a desire to eat less food during their next meal, than they did after consuming an olive oil look alike placebo. They verified this effect in people with capsules containing a concentrated form of the oil (pinolenic acid) in a product called Pinno Thin. Remember, one tablespoon of pine nuts is equal to about one fat serving and about 60 calories.

IODINE

Too Much Iodine

The fear of radiation traveling to this country from the damaged Japanese Nuclear Power plants in 2011 had many of my patients rushing to buy iodine supplements, despite pleas from health officials that it was not necessary and could be dangerous. Side effects are seen in as many as 8% of those given potassium iodide, including swelling of the lips and face (angioedema-allergic reactions including hives and death), severe bleeding and bruising, fever, skin rashes, swollen salivary glands with increased salivation, a metallic/brassy taste in the mouth, a sense of burning in the mouth and throat, headaches, soreness in the teeth and gums, stomach discomfort, diarrhea, joint pain, and lymph node enlargement.

Radioactive Iodine

When given in a crisis to those directly exposed to radiation, potassium iodide blocks the radioactive uptake that can cause thyroid cancer. In 1986, the winds after the Chernobyl nuclear reactor melt down carried the radioactive iodine downwind to Belarus and Ukraine. They were given no protection and had a hundred fold increase in thyroid cancers; but in Poland, potassium iodine was handed out and there was no increase in thyroid cancer. Late radioactive exposure in the majority of the Russian people after Chernobyl was from drinking the local cow's milk, eating fish and wild herbs (from grass eaten and carried far and wide by wild boars).

What Is The Iodine Dose That Is Safe?

For children and adults the Recommended Dietary Amounts (RDA) are: children 1 to 8 years, 90 micrograms (mcg) per day; 9 to 13 years, 120 mcg per day; people age 14 and older, 150 mcg per day. NOT 130 milligrams (mg) used for radiation poisoning (not prevention).

Our Bodies Need Iodine

Iodine (chemical symbol I, atomic number 53) is a nonmetal that belongs to a group of chemical elements known as halogens (elements with 7 electrons in their outer shell). Fluoride, chlorine, bromide and iodine are in this group. Iodine is the smallest and most reactive element in the halogen family. Our bodies need iodine but cannot make it. The needed iodine must come from our diet. There is very little iodine in food, unless it has been added during processing (i.e., salt). Most of the world's iodine is found in the ocean, where it is concentrated by sea life, especially deep water fish like cod and halibut, and in seaweed.

Thyroid Dysfunction

The thyroid gland needs iodine to make hormones. If the thyroid doesn't have enough iodine to do its job, God made feedback systems from the pituitary to produce Thyroid Stimulating Hormone (TSH), which causes the thyroid to work harder. This can cause a swollen neck from an enlarged thyroid gland. The most recognized form of iodine deficiency is a goiter. Iodine deficiency and the resulting low levels of thyroid hormone can cause generalized fatigue and women to stop ovulating, leading to infertility. Iodine deficiency can also lead to an autoimmune (body attacking itself) disease of the thyroid and may increase the risk of getting thyroid cancer. Taking small amounts of iodine orally can improve thyroid storm, hypothyroidism, and goiters.

Iodine Deficiencies

Around the world, iodine deficiency is thought to be the most common preventable cause of mental retardation. Iodine is depleted by a high fat diet. In iodine deficiency, taking iodine supplements can kill fungus, bacteria, and other microorganisms such as amoebas. It is also used for treating a skin disease caused by a fungus, cutaneous sporotrichosis (Rose gardener's disease). It has been used for fibrocystic disease of the breasts, cystic ovaries, and restless leg syndrome. Some researchers, including me, think that iodine deficiency might also increase the risk of other cancers such as prostate, breast, endometrial, and ovarian cancer. Countries with high iodine intakes, like Japan and Greenland, had the same incidence of cancer detection as the rest of the world, but interestingly the cancer cells did not spread pass the basement membranes. Therefore, deaths from these cancers were very low. Increased dietary iodine intake appears to be the correlating factor.

These Medicines And Iodine Don't Mix

Amiodarone: (Cordarone) is used for cardiac dysrrthymias and contains iodine. Taking iodine supplements along with amiodarone (Cordarone) might cause too much iodine in your blood.

Lithium: Large amounts of iodine can decrease thyroid function. Lithium can increase iodine's effects on the thyroid.

Medications for high blood pressure: (ACE inhibitors) and Angiotensin receptor blockers (ARBs). Some medications for high blood pressure might decrease how quickly the body gets rid of potassium. Most iodide supplements contain potassium. Taking potassium iodide along with some medications for high blood pressure might cause too much potassium in the body. ACEs include: captopril (Capoten), enalapril (Vasotec), lisinopril (Prinivil, Zestril), ramipril (Altace). ARBs include: losartan (Cozaar), valsartan (Diovan), irbesartan (Avapro), candesartan (Atacand), Benicar (olmesartan), telmisartan (Micardis), and eprosartan (Teveten).

Water pills: (Potassium-sparing diuretics) Most iodine supplements contain potassium. Some "water pills" might also increase potassium in the body. Taking potassium iodide along with some "water pills" might cause too much potassium to be in the body. Some "water pills" that increase potassium in the body include spironolactone (Aldactone), triamterene (Dyrenium), Dyazide/Maxide and amiloride (Midamor).

Iodine Containing Foods

Iodized Salt	100 grams	3000 mcg
Cereals and Breads	100 grams	10-11 mcg
Meat	100 grams	26-27 mcg
Vegetables	100 grams	32-33 mcg

Food	Amount	Iodine
Fruits	100 grams	4-5 mcg
Malt bread	100 grams	29-30 mcg
Jaffa cakes	100 grams	More than 32 mcg
Naan Bread	100 grams	28-29 mcg
Mayonnaise	100 grams	35-36 mcg
Boiled Egg	1 egg	23.76 mcg
Low Fat Yogurt	1 cup	87 mcg
Strawberries	1 cup	13 mcg
Kelp*	0.25 cup	415 mcg
Cow's Milk (2%)	1 cup	58-59 mcg
Gouda Cheese	40 grams	13.6 mcg
Ice Cream	45-50 grams	9.6-9.7 mcg
Cheddar Cheese	1 ounce	5-20 mcg
Cottage Cheese	1/2 cup with around 2% milk fat	25-70 mcg

*Dulse (red seaweed), Kombu (Chinese kelp), Arame (Japanese seaweed), Wakame (brown seaweed), Hijike (seaweed leaf), Nori (green seaweed used in sushi).

References:

Marine, D., *"Prevention and Treatment of Simple Goiter (with iodine),"* Atl. Med J. 26:437-442:1923.

Abraham, G., *"Ortho-iodo-supplementation: Iodine Sufficiency of The Whole Human Body,"* Optimax Research Corp., Torrance, CA

en.wikipedia.org/wiki/Iodine

www.nlm.nih.gov/medlineplus/druginfo/natural/35.html

RADIATION INDUCED CANCERS

- What Chance Do I Have Of Getting Cancer?

I am continually asked what the likelihood is of developing radiation induced cancer, in light of the nuclear disaster in Japan, 2011. Radiation consists of several types of subatomic particles, principally those called gamma rays, neutrons, electrons, and alpha particles, that shoot through space at very high speeds (approximately 100,000 miles per second). They easily damage your cells and if not quickly repaired can cause a fatal cancer to develop, or if it occurs in reproductive cells, it can cause genetic defects in later generations of offspring. So is being struck by a particle of radiation a serious event?

Cancer Death

There are well documented cases of radiation induced cancer in humans. The most common cause of death in the U.S. is cancer, accounting currently for one out every two deaths. Radiation may mutate your DNA in a few cells when they are dividing and some may form cancer cells. This occurs every moment of your life, but a healthy immune system (good nutrition) will recognize, attack and destroy the cancerous cells before starting a deadly growth cycle. We are constantly bombarded with radiation that disrupts our cell's DNA. We are pelted with 15,000 of these particles of radiation every second of our life. These particles, totaling 500 billion per year, or 40 trillion in a lifetime, are from natural sources. In addition, radiation from medical X-rays add to this bewildering assault on our bodies (a typical X-ray bombards us with over a trillion particles of radiation). Are all cancers caused by radiation exposure 10 to 30 years earlier? No, about 1% of cancers have been traced to radiation exposure!

Leukemia

The early scientists who worked with x-rays and radioactive substances did not realize the risk. Many died from skin, bone cancer and leukemia. Leukemia is a disease characterized by a great excess of immature white cells in the blood and can be likened to a blood cancer. Marie Curie, for example, who first isolated radium from uranium ore, died of leukemia (aged 67;1934) as did her daughter, Irene-assistant (aged 56; 1956), (Marie's husband died in a horse drawn carriage traffic accident-age 47;1906).

Radium Induced Bone Cancer

In the 1920's, watch dials were painted with a radium based luminous paint. The employees, all women, who did this work often licked their paint brushes to give them a sharp point and ingested a small quantity of the paint each time they did this. The radium in the paint collected in their bones and resulted in bone tumors 8 to 40 years later.

Nuclear Radiation Exposure

The largest number of human beings exposed to high levels of whole body radiation are the survivors of the Hiroshima (August 6, 1945) and Nagasaki (August 9, 1945) atom bomb attacks. Nearly 80,000 of these people have been carefully studied in the years since the war. Of survivors, 126 died of leukemia. This is nearly double the normal figure for this number of people. The incidence of leukemia was related to the distance from the explosion and therefore to the radiation dose received.

The highest incidence was in those survivors closest to the explosion. This provided clear evidence of the dose dependent relationship of leukemia to radiation, i.e. the higher the dose, the greater the risk. The study of these survivors also showed an increase in stomach, lung and breast cancers. These have taken much longer to develop and some were just appearing in the year 2000.

Thyroid Cancer

Radioactive Iodine-131 (I-131) has a decay half life of about eight days of both beta and gamma emissions. This is the predominate radiation leaked from the Japanese nuclear power plants. Due to its mode of beta decay, I-131 is notable for causing mutation and death in cells which it penetrates, and other cells up to several millimeters away. Iodine in food is absorbed and preferentially concentrated in the thyroid where it is needed for its functioning. When I-131 is present in high levels in the environment from radioactive fallout, it can be absorbed through contaminated food, and will also accumulate in the thyroid. As it decays, it may cause damage to the thyroid. The primary risk from exposure to high levels of I-131 is the chance occurrence of radiogenic thyroid cancer in later life. Other risks include the possibility of non-cancerous growths and thyroiditis. In medicine years ago, it was not uncommon to irradiate the thyroid area in childhood. This caused an increased risk of thyroid cancer, which has been recognized for over 50 years. Studies of the effects of external radiation (airport scanning), medical diagnostic I-131 use, environmental radioactive iodine (natural sources and nuclear power leaks) and gamma-ray (X-ray) exposure have demonstrated the risks of radiation exposure and thyroid carcinomas. These studies show a paradox, in that the risk of thyroid cancer is increased with exposure to low or moderate levels of external radiation. However, thyroid cancer risks are much lower after high level irradiation that results in thyroid cell death or reduced capacity of cells to divide.

Radon Exposure

Those of use living in the mountains of Western North Carolina (and other radon hot spots around the world) are much more likely to die from lung cancer from radon exposure in our granite rocks under our homes then from a tiny bite of radioactive material drifting over use from Japan. So what do I recommend? Be vigilant and pray without ceasing!

References:

The Management of Graves' Disease in Children, with Special Emphasis on Radioiodine Treatment. Scott A. Rivkees, Charles Sklar and Michael Freemark J. Clin. Endocrinol. Metab. 1998 83: 3767-3776

en.wikipedia.org/wiki/Thyroid_cancer
http://www.phyast.pitt.edu/~blc/book/chapter5.html
http://www.cancer.org/cancer/cancercauses/othercarcinogens/medicaltreatments/radiation-exposure-and-cancer

ALCOHOL AND THE CHRISTIAN

The Medical Literature

Researchers have found antioxidants, such as flavonoids and a substance called resveratrol, have heart-healthy benefits. These antioxidants are found under the skin of the grape, not in the alcohol as some alcoholic-loving scientists had hoped. Alcohol is associated with:

1) hypertension,
2) cardiac dysrrhythmias (irregular heart beats) including atrial fibrillation,
3) congestive cardiomyopathy (weakened heart muscle),
4) bleeding stroke in young people (Am J Psych 148:3, 296, 3/91 and Honolulu Heart Program-JAMA vol.255, no.17, 2311-14, 5/2/86),
5) cirrhosis of the liver (fibrosis),
6) bleeding ulcers and esophagus,
7) osteoporosis,
8) psychosis
9) sudden death,
10) impairment in cardiac performance (decreased blood pumped) can be elicited in normal persons who consume 4 oz of Canadian whiskey. (Cardiology product news 10/83)
11) loss of brain tissue in chronic alcoholics causes decrease cerebral blood flow and is associated with dementia. Some increase of blood flow and return of cognitive function is seen with abstinence. (Am J Psych 148:3, 292-305, 1991)
12) reports of alcohol reducing heart disease is from the difference in diet not the alcohol.
13) 14,000 women studied over 40 years old, who had 2 drinks a day were 50% more likely to get breast cancer.
14) deaths in the US-100,000/yr (includes traffic accidents)

15) nitrosamines from beer act to increase rectal cancer in men and women, 1.73 and 1.55 times normal, respectively. (Am J. Epi 134:157-66, 91)
16) producing muscle damage in healthy human volunteers. (Science vol.175, 327-28, 1/21/72)
17) known since 1785 published reports, that alcohol predisposes to infection and increases it severity by interfering with the normal immune host defense mechanisms. (JAMA vol.256, no.11, 1474-79, 9/19/86)
18) causing worsening blood sugars (higher) in the elderly. (Internal medicine and Cardiology news 8/15/92)
19) fetal alcohol syndrome (FAS) (JAMA vol.245, no.23, 2436-39, 6/19/81) seen in about 1 on 600 births (clear cut cases counted only) in U.S., Sweden and France.
20) prenatal and postnatal growth impairment. Children are usually below the third percentile for height and weight. Men with FAS usually are 5'2.5" to 5'6" in height.
21) central nervous system (CNS) dysfunction. The first sign is microcephaly (small head). Hyperactivity, especially of the fine motor movement, is seen in older children. Retardation of IQ (60 to 75) is reported in severe cases. Intelligence could not be improved with improved home and social environment! (Alcoholism 2:165-170, 1978)
22) FLK (medical term for particular facial pattern, "Funny Looking Kid")
23) major organ system malformations
24) miscarriage twice as high in women who have as little as 2 drinks a week. (Lancet 2:176-180, 1980)
25) testosterone (male hormone) being converted to estradiol (female hormone). This occurred with as few as 3 drinks/wk. (Alcoholism: Clin and Exp Res, vol.16, no.1, 87-92, 7/92)

Wise Counsel

Ill effects of alcohol (Prov 23:29-30; 20:1;Hab 2:5; Lev 10:11; Ez 44:23):

The nervous system weakened and mind beclouded. "Christ is seeking to save, and Satan to destroy. I ask you that have reasoning powers to think on these things. The man that is intoxicated is robbed of his reason. Satan comes in and takes possession of him and imbues him with his spirit; and his first desire is to bruise or kill some of his loved ones. Yet men will allow this accursed thing to go on, that makes man lower than the beast. What has the drunkard obtained? Nothing but a madman's brain." Temperance. 288

Gastritis "The inflamed condition of the drunkard's stomach is often pictured as illustrating the effect of alcoholic liquors." Ministry of Healing, 325

They Have Sold Their Will Power. "There is in the world a multitude of degraded human beings, who have, by yielding in their youth to the temptation to use tobacco and alcohol, poisoned the tissues of the human structure, and perverted their reasoning powers, until the result is just as Satan meant it to be. The faculties of thought are clouded. The victims yield to the temptation for alcohol, and they sell what reason they have for a glass of liquor." Temperance, 36

Lives Are Sacrificed. "Alcohol and tobacco pollute the blood of men, and thousands of lives are yearly sacrificed to these poisons." The Health Reformer, November, 1871

Nature of Crimes Committed Under Alcohol. "The result of liquor drinking is demonstrated by the awful murders that take place. How often it is found that theft, incendiarism, murder, were committed under the influence of liquor. Yet the liquor curse is legalized, and works untold ruin in the hands of those who love to tamper with that which ruins not only the poor victim, but his whole family." The Review and Herald, May 1, 1900 (Counsels On Diet, 436-7).

Violation of God's Law. "Why do not those who have excellent reasoning powers reason from cause to effect? Why do they not advocate reform by planting their feet firmly on principle, determined not to taste alcoholic drink or to use tobacco? These are poisons, and their use is a violation of God's law. Some say, when an effort is made to enlighten them on this point, I will leave off by degrees. But Satan laughs at all such decisions. He says, They are secure in my power. I have no fear of them on that ground." Temperance, 103

Legacy of disease and imbecility transmitted to offspring. "What a record will appear when the accounts of life are balanced in the book of God! It will then appear that vast sums of money have been expended for tobacco and alcoholic liquors! For what? To ensure health and prolong life? Oh, no! To aid in the perfection of Christian character and a fitness for the society of holy angels? Oh, no! But to minister to a depraved, unnatural appetite for that which poisons and kills not only the user but those to whom he transmits his legacy of disease and imbecility. —The Signs of the Times, October 27, 1887 (Temperance, 66).

Biblical Proof-No Alcohol

Does the Bible contradict itself?

1. Verses against the use of fermented wine: Lev 10:8-11; Jud 13:3,4; Prov 31:4,5; 23:31; 20:1; Hab 2:5; Eph 5:18; 1Tim 3:2,3
2. Verses for the use of "wine": Gen 27:28; 49:10-12; Ps 104:14,15; Isa 55:1; Am 9:13; Jn 2:10.11.

Pro Wine Theory

This view is held by most Christian churches. They say the Bible speaks only of fermented wine. Therefore, any condemnation of wine refers not to the kind of wine (alcoholic), but to the amount consumed. Wine (English), vinum (Latin), oinos (Greek), and yayin (Hebrew) have historically been used to refer to the juice of the grape-fermented or not. Therefore, the context and verse by verse consistency of the Bible is required for a proof.

In the Septuagint Inter-Testamental Greek Old Testament the Hebrew word for fresh grape juice (tirosh) is 33 times translated oinos (wine) without the word "new" correctly added. Most translators, it is believed, because of their predilection for drinking have chosen to continue to modify the original intent.

Matt 9:17 New Wine In New Wineskins

No fresh/new goatskin pouches/jars could hold together from the pressure of fermenting new wine. The common practice of the day was to squeeze out the wine from a press, strain it, boil it and immediately place it into fresh wineskins to insure the absence of fermenting substances. Old skins had albuminoid matter adhering to the skin which set up fermentation/gas production. This understanding makes the symbolism clear. New wine in new wineskins represent regeneration. Old wine symbolizes corruption and old wineskins are our sinful nature before conversion. The new wine of the gospel could not be put in them!

Most mistakenly believe that it was impossible to keep grape juice from fermenting 2000 years ago before refrigeration. But contrary to popular assumptions it was harder to keep alcoholic wine from becoming acidic, moldy or foul tasting than it was to keep grape juice fresh. You had to add salt, sea-water, liquid or solid pitch, boiled-down grape pulp, marble dust, lime, sulfur fumes or crushed iris to keep alcoholic wine from spoiling; all of which added an undesirable taste.

Ancient sources (non-biblical; including Aristotle 384-322 B.C, Athenaeus 280 A.D., Pliny 24-79 A.D.) give 4 ways of preventing fermentation of fresh grape juice.

1) boiling down to syrup.
2) separating fermentable pulp from juice by filtration.
3) placing freshly pressed juice in sealed leather bottles/jars with immersion in cold pond water.
4) fumigating jars with sulphur acid before sealing them.

Prov 31:4 ... It Is Not For Kings To Drink Wine (Yayin)...

This text does not say "it is not for kings to drink much wine"; but it is a prohibition-none.

Jesus And The Cana Wedding - Desire Of Ages 144

Many believe that the "good" wine in Jn 2:10 was good because of its high alcohol content. Here are their reasons:

A) This was a spring passover wedding (Jn 2:13), therefore 6 months from the last grape harvest, thus the grape juice had to be fermented.

B) The master of the banquet describes fermented wine that Jesus made. In Roman times the best wine was grape juice. Pliny-"wines are most beneficial when all their potency has been removed by the strainer." Plutarch-wine is "much more pleasant to drink" when it "neither inflames the brain nor infests the mind or passions" because its strength has been removed through frequent filtering. Rabbi S. M. Isaac (Eminent 19th century editor of *The Jewish Messenger*) - "The Jews do not, in their feasts for sacred purposes, including the marriage feast, ever use any kind of fermented drinks."

C) "Well drunk" means intoxicated. Greek word "well drunk" (methusko) can also mean to drink freely-RSV, or sense of satiety. Many still insist that Jesus provided a better quality, alcoholic wine (believed to be 120-180 gallons), therefore they must conclude that Jesus miraculously made a large additional quantity of intoxicating wine in order that the wedding party could continue its reckless indulgence. Moral consistency demands that Christ then be responsible for their intoxication. Scripturally and morally Christ produced fresh grape juice--"the good wine." The very adjective used to describe the wine (kalos), that we in English translate "good" denotes moral excellence. The Greek word "agathos" which simply means good is not used.

The Communion Wine

Fundamentalist Christians believe that Christ not only used "alcoholic wine" but commanded it be used until the end of time as a memorial of his redeeming blood (Mt 26:28-29; Mk 14:24-25).

A) "Fruit of the vine" was *allegedly* equivalent to fermented wine.

The noun "fruit" (gennema) means-that which is produced in a natural state, just as gathered. Fermented wine is in a unnatural form of the fruit-a form of decay. The Jewish historian Josephus (contemporary of the apostles) uses this same phrase "the fruit of the vine" to mean sweet, unfermented juice in his writings.

B) "All" to drink the cup.

It is unlikely that Christ said drink ye all the Lord's Supper alcoholic wine. The usual Passover cup of wine was 3/4 pint (12 oz). There are some whom the simple taste or smell of alcohol is medically harmful. Could Christ after teaching us to pray "lead us not into temptation" have made a place of irresistible temptation for some and danger for all?

C) The law of fermentation.

The mosaic law required the exclusion of all fermented articles during Passover (ex 12:15; 13:6,7). Fermented wine stands for human depravity and divine indignation (this symbolism is all through Revelation). The bread during communion is to be unleaven-to represent perfect Christ's body, a pure atonement for our sins. Leaven = corrupt nature, Christ knew this definition in calling Pharisees "the leaven" (Mt 16:12). In the wine, Christ's blood is to represent the incorruptible. It does not make sense to have unleaven bread and fermented wine as symbols when they mean the opposite. Thus, a fitting emblem is pure grape juice to mean Christ's untainted blood shed for the remission of our sins.

In summary, Christians are a "Royal Priesthood" (1Pe 2:9) called to "keep sane and sober" (1Pe 4:7). 1 Pe 1:13's best translation (nephontes teleios) -be completely or perfectly abstinent.

Bacchiocchi, S., *"Wine in the Bible: A Biblical Study On The Use Of Alcoholic Beverages."* Biblicalperpectives.com Taken from and expanded by Royce Bailey MD, MPH, March 5, 1993.

White, E.G., Spirit of Prophecy Books. Last updated May 27, 2010.

ALZHEIMER'S DISEASE
REDUCE YOUR DNA DAMAGE
- Make Dried Fruit A Habit

Alzheimer's Disease (AD):

Estimates provided by the National Alzheimer's Association indicate that 10% of the population over the age of 65 has AD and almost 50% of the population over the age of 85 have AD. People with AD live three to 20 years from the time of diagnosis. NC Med J. Jan/Feb 2005, vol 66, number 1:14.

Oxygen Radical Absorbance Capacity (or AC)

The anti-oxidant effect of raisins (like dried plums/prunes) has a high Oxygen Radical Absorbance Capacity (ORAC). Simply, they have a strong ability to neutralize free radicals, reversing our bodies tendency to "rust" out. Athletes competing in triathlons who were given raisins before competition had increased antioxidant levels in their bloodstream within 15 to 30 minutes. After 60 minutes, the antioxidants had moved from the blood stream into various tissues of the athletes' bodies. Eating dried fruit before undertaking any type of strenuous activity can help prevent oxidative stress; in other words, stress induced DNA damage. This is the same type of damage associated with tissue aging, memory loss and loss of brain function. – Gene Spiller, Stanford University, presentation at the 43rd Annual American College of Nutrition.

Dried Plums

Using the Nutritional Density Index, we can compare dried fruit to fresh fruit.

Ounce for ounce DRIED PLUMS have:

Antioxidants (Vitamin A&E) = 16x bananas

Help slow the aging process and help protect your cells from cancer causing "free radicals"

Potassium = 8x apples

Helps maintain healthy blood pressure and promotes muscle energy.

Vitamin B = 6x oranges

Supports your nervous system, skin and eyes. It helps in the formation of antibodies.

Vitamin K = 83x bananas

Helps protect against heart disease and osteoporosis. It helps regulates your blood sugar, slows aging and helps clotting factors.

Dietary Fiber = 5x apples

Necessary for digestive health and helps fight heart disease, diabetes and cancer.

NO Cholesterol

Has protein and carbohydrates but no cholesterol.

Low in sodium

Can be eaten on a salt restricted diet.

Diabetic Exchange: 1½ fruit

For Your Snack Attack Try Dried Fruits

Everybody knows fruit is good for them. We just need to get into a habit of eating more antioxidant foods, like prunes and raisins. Next time you're searching for a snack, keep in mind that just a handful of these dried fruits can pack a very powerful punch when it comes to helping you stay healthy by preventing DNA damage to our bodies and thus helping prevent AD.

Note: Try to limit sulfur containing dried fruit.

PROSTATE HEALTH

BPH/Prostate Cancer Causes

Benign prostatic hypertrophy (BPH) or enlarged prostate gland affects more than 60% of men ages 50 to 60. When sleep is disrupted from frequent trips to the bathroom at night with little to show for it, it is time to seek treatment for your BPH. This is because of progressive prostate enlargement obstructing the outflow of urine from your bladder. Testosterone is converted to dihydrotestosterone (DHT), which binds to the prostate tissue and causes it to abnormally enlarge. Remember, symptoms of BPH are similar to early cancer of the prostate symptoms.

1. Obesity increases prostate cancer risk 2.5 times above normal. Men who have had prostate surgery who were obese at ages 25 to 40 or gained a lot of weight between the ages of 25 and the diagnosis of cancer, were twice as likely to have a five year recurrence then non obese men.-Clinical Cancer Research, October 2005.

2. Heavy smoking doubles the risk of aggressive prostate cancer compared to those that never smoked. Said another way; men underage 65 with a cigarette smoking history of 40 or more pack/years face a 100% increase risk of getting a lethal form of cancer. – Fred Hutchinson

Cancer Research Center, Aug 3, 2003

3. Breast and prostate cancers are linked to consumption of dairy products. Insulin-like growth factor (IGF-1) is found in cow's milk and is increased in the blood of individuals consuming dairy products on a regular basis. Cow's IGF-1 and human's IGF-1 is identical, so your body just -- plug and play. Other nutrients that increase IGF-1 are also found in cow's milk. Men with the highest levels of IGF-1 had four times the risk of prostate cancer compared with those with the lowest levels. -Science 1998;279:563-5

Navaho Indians Had No Cancer Except...

There was only one person to get prostate cancer among the 5,000 Navaho Indians in San Juan County, Utah between 1950 and 1985. This Navaho was the only Indian to raise chickens and eat eggs. (Navaho's have a taboo about birds–a fearful reverence). Chickens have an extremely high cancer incidence. The 'carcinogen' in chickens is avian leukosis virus, a close relative of HIV (AIDS). It was discovered in 1911 by Rous and is passed in eggs. Be warned about eating raw or over easy eggs, for it may cause prostate cancer. -Internal Medicine News, Feb 15, 1992.

Adventist Health Study 1980

6763 white male Seventh-day Adventists were studied between 1960 and 1980. The dead ones showed us that overweight men had a significantly higher risk of fatal prostate cancer (2.5 times more) then men near their desirable weight. Dietary associations were seen in fatal prostate cancer in the consumption of milk (ice cream), cheese, eggs and meat. There was an orderly dose-response between each of the four animal products and the risk. The risk of fatal prostate cancer was 3.6 times higher for those that heavily consumed all four animal products. Thus, the Adventist Health Study suggests that consumption of animal products and obesity are risk factors for fatal prostate cancer. -Am J Epi 1984;120:244-250.

Physician Health Study 2001

20,885 men in the Physician's Health Study over 11 years found 1,012 cases of prostate cancer. Those with the highest dairy product and calcium intake had a 30% increased risk of prostate cancer. Each additional 500 mg of calcium from diary products taken each day increased the risk of prostate cancer by 16% (P = 0.03). The higher the dairy calcium intake, the lower the vitamin D levels [1, 25 (OH) 2D3] in the blood. Vitamin D hormone protects against prostate cancer. As I've said before, milk should not be a source for your calcium. It doesn't help your bones and increases your risk for glandular (adenocarcinoma) cancer (breast, colon and prostate). -Am J Clin Nutr 2001;74:549-554.

What Should We Do?

"Let the diet reform be progressive. Let the people be taught how to prepare food without the use of milk or butter. Tell them that the time will soon come when there will be no safety in using eggs. Milk, cream, or butter, because disease in animals is increasing in proportion to the increase of wickedness among men. The time is near when, because of the iniquity of the fallen race, the whole animal creation will groan under the diseases that curse our earth.

God will give His people ability and tact to prepare wholesome food without these recipes. Let the people discard all unwholesome recipes. Let them learn how to live healthfully, teaching to others what they have learned. Let them impart this knowledge as they would Bible instruction. Let them teach the people to preserve the health and increase the strength by avoiding the large amount of cooking that has filled the world with chronic invalids. By precept and example make it plain that the food which God gave Adam in his sinless state is the best for man's use as he seeks to regain that sinless state." How did she know that? Testimonies to the Church, vol.7; 1902:132-137 and Counsels on Health: 478-479.

Treatments For BPH: Prostatectomy

Prostatectomy, or removal of prostate tissue, (the reem job) is very effective in relieving most of the symptoms of BPH. 33% of all males in the US have undergone surgical removal of their prostate gland by the time they are 85 years old.

Saw Palmetto

Serenoa repens (saw palmetto) is an extract from the berry of a small palm tree (South Carolina state tree; the tree is even on their flag). Saw Palmetto prevents the formation of dihydrotestosterone (DHT) by blocking an enzyme and by inhibiting DHT binding to hormone receptors on the prostate cells. Take 162 mg twice a day of a standardized saw palmetto extract of 85% fatty acids and sterols (the active ingredients). 18 studies with 3000 men found saw palmetto just as effective as prescription meds in reducing BPH symptoms.-*Benefits of Saw Palmetto Reviewed, JAMA, 1999.*

Pygeum

Pygeum africanum is a large evergreen tree native to central and southern Africa. Pygeum inhibits the production of dihydrotestosterone (DHT). 100 mg a day of standardized extract (containing 14% terpenesand sterols and 0.5% ferulic acids) can reduce the symptoms of urgency and painful urination caused by an enlarged prostate (BPH) by 46%. It works better when combined with 320 mg/day of saw palmetto. It can take up to six weeks to see results as opposed to prescription BPH meds (cardura/doxazosin, hytrin or uroxatral/quinazoline, flomax/ tamsulosin).In large doses pygeum can cause intestinal irritation such as nausea and stomach pain.-*Urology, Sept 1999*.

Zinc

Zinc deficiency has been linked not only to prostatitis (inflammation of the prostate gland) but also to BPH. A hand full of pumpkin seeds (1/4 cup-126 calories) supplies 20% of your daily zinc requirement. Taking too much zinc (more than 100 mg a day) increases the risk of advanced prostate cancer. -*J Natl Cancer Inst, July 2003*.

Isoflavones: More Soy And Beans

Countries that eat more soy and other legumes (red, green, black and other beans) have prostate cancers occur later in life and it grows more slowly. Isoflavones (genostein, diadzein, biochanin A and formononetin) found in many beans are weakly estrogenic. Isoflavones can block estrogen like compounds in our environment in the forms of plastics, pesticides and other synthetic compounds. Genistein, best known from soy but found in most beans, reduced the proliferation of prostate tumors. Biochanin A inhibits the growth of prostate cancer cells. Sources of isoflavones should come from the natural source and not from a pill. The recommendation is 45 mg a day of isoflavones in a variety of foods. -*"Isoflavones And The Prevention And Treatment Of Prostate Disease: Is There A Role?" Cleveland Clin J Med, March 2003;70:203-216*.

Vitamin E

Multiple studies have not found a benefit in taking vitamin E, in cancer or cardiovascular health. Full vitamin E (tocotrienols andtocopherols - all eight parts) caused cancer cell growth and the ability to form new cells to decrease by 50%. Get your vitamin E in seeds. A hand full of sunflower or pumpkin seeds per day is a good natural source of vitamin E. Another good source is peanuts.

Lycopene

Bright red carotenoid phytochemical, lycopene, found in tomatoes, watermelon and pink grapefruit, may prevent macular degeneration, sun damage to the skin, cancer, and even osteoporosis. Lycopene in the pill form is ten times more effective than vitamin E at preventing malignant cell transformations of the prostate, cervix and GI tract. Absorption of lycopene is better in cooked tomatoes, than in fresh, and still better when you add a little olive oil to your tomato sauce. Dietary protection of cancer and cardiovascular health is found in 3 mg of lycopene (100 gm of fresh or cooked tomatoes/about 1/5 of a pound). Watermelon has more lycopene than tomatoes (½ cup of cubed watermelon). 20 mg of lycopene a day is recommended for treatment of BPH. Eating 3/4 cup of tomato sauce a day (30 mg lycopene) can cut your risk of exercise induced asthma in half. *-Letsliveonline.com, June 2004:28.-Men's Health, May 2001:34.*

Selenium

Men with the greatest selenium (Se) intake from natural sources had about a 66% lower risk of developing advanced prostate cancer over the next decade than those that had a lower intake amount. This is because selenium is known to interfere with binding of the toxic trace mineral cadmium (Cd). Cadmium stimulates the growth of prostate epithelial cells and their malignant transformations. Cadmium is found in many foods, in drinking water, and in the environment. Your Se/Cd ratio may predict your chance of prostate cancer in the future. Selenium is found in seeds and nutritional (brewer's) yeast. Recommended 200 mcg of selenium a day. *-Natl Cancer Inst, 1998; 90 (16):1219-24-Biological Trace Elements Research, Feb 2005;103, 2:103-108.*

Omega-3

Flaxseed, a source of omega-3 fatty acids (alpha linolenic acid-ALA), and lignan have been shown to inhibit melanoma, breast cancer and prostate cancer growth. Two tablespoons of freshly ground flaxseed a day decreased free testosterone and cholesterol levels, by day 2143. Low grade prostate disease had a decreased cell proliferation in the flaxseed groups, but a recent study of 47,000 men showed that flaxseed oil may worsen advanced prostate cancer. The reason was high levels of ALA did not convert to the beneficial EPA/DHA Omega-3. EPA (eicosapentaenoic acid) and DHA (docosahexaenoic acid) are polyunsaturated fatty acids that are part of the Omega-3 family and found in cold water fish. The enzyme delta six desaturase converts ALA to EPA/DHA, but delta six desaturase is severely inhibited by elevated insulin levels. Thus, anyone with diabetes type 2, that is over weight, having high cholesterol or high blood pressure can have elevated insulin levels and should not take flax seed oil for their prostate! *-Am J Clin Nutr, July 2004;80(1):204-216.*

Buchu Leaf

Barosma betulina has a pungent aroma, due to its highly volatile oils. Buchu's actions are mostly anti-inflammatory, diuretic and antiseptic. It is effective in the treatment of painful urination, kidney/bladder inflammations and infections and "irritable bladder." Buchu is very soothing to the pelvic nerves. Take 100 mg to 300 mg a day.

Couch Grass Root

Agropyron repens helps reduce uncontrollable urination, pain and burning. Couch grass is loaded with carotene, potassium and vitamin C. Take 100 mg to 300 mg a day or as a tea. Avoid couch grass if you have blood in your urine. Use Horsetail or South African Star Grass extract instead.

Beta-Sistosterol

Take phytosterols (plant sterols) to reduce urinary symptoms associated with BPH. It is found in all plants, but is in the highest amounts in seeds, beans and grains. Recommended dose is 20 mg a day.

Statins

Cholesterol reducing statin drugs lowered the risk of prostate cancer by 62%. *-Am J Epidemiol 2005;162:318-325.*

Indian Frankincense

Boswellia serrata is a gum resin of a tree native to India. It inhibits prostate cancer by blocking the conversion of arachidonic acid toprostaglandin E2 and 5-HETE. It also down regulates tumor necrosisfactor alpha (TNF-a) to normal. Recommended 400 mg of standardized boswellia extract (containing 60% boswellic acid) three times a day.

Garlic

Both fresh and garlic supplements prevent prostate cancer by interfering with the initiation and promotion phases, and by blocking arachidonic acid metabolism. The quality of garlic varies, so choose a standardized extract or the real thing. Two fresh cloves a day for cancer patients.

Stinging Nettles

Urtica dioica is used as a first line in the treatment of BPH in Germany. There are over fifty compounds in stinging nettle. Stinging nettles works by blocking the effect of estrogen and free androgen, thus lowering the serum estrogen levels, reducing inflammation. Recommended dose is 600-1, 200 mg of a 5:1 extract or 120 mg twice a day of a 10:1 extract (standardized amino acid content). Some people are allergic to stinging nettle and it can cause stomach upset.

Turmeric (Curcumin)

Curcuma longa is the major ingredient of curry powder. Turmeric inhibits prostate cancer by blocking the conversion of arachidonic acid to prostaglandin E2 and 5-HETE, by inducing cell death and regulating the tumor suppressor gene p53. Recommended 400-600 mg three times a day. It works great for arthritis too. This is a spice and can cause stomach upset.-*"Therapeutic Potential Of Curcumin In Human Prostate Cancer. II*

Curcumin Inhibits Tyrosine Kinase Activity Of Epidermal Growth Factor Receptor and Depletes The Protein," Mol Urol, Spring 2000;4(1):1-6.

B12 AND YOUR HEALTH

The vitamin, B12 (Cyanocobalamin), was discovered in 1948. It is a water soluble vitamin, so you need a regular supply; because it is water soluble it is unlikely for you to over dose on it. Vitamin B12 helps maintain healthy nerve cells, normal electrical function of the body's synapses and robust red blood cells (improving oxygen and CO_2 carrying capacity). It is also needed to help make DNA and RNA, the genetic material in all our cells. Vitamin B12 contains the metal cobalt, thus the name cobalamin.

Where Is B12 Found?

It is found in nuts, seeds, potato skins, nutritional (brewer's) yeast, B12 fortified foods (breads, breakfast cereals) and animal products. B12 can be found in fermented soybean products such as tempeh, natto, and miso; in single cell micro-organisms such as algae, Spirulina and Chlorella; and in seaweed products. It is very rare to see B12 deficiency in 3rd world countries, despite their restricted diets.

Symptoms Of B12 Deficiency

Signs, symptoms, and health problems associated with vitamin B12 deficiency can be a common cause of pernicious anemia, sprue, disorders of blood (macrocytic anemia-red cells are too large and the bone marrow can not make enough red cells), nerve damage, fatigue, light-headedness, change in appetite, nausea, bleeding gums, soreness of the mouth or tongue, constipation or diarrhea. B12 deficiency has been misdiagnosed as fibromyalgia, and has been implicated in a spectrum of neuropsychiatric disorders (mood swings, depression, irritability, psychosis, dementia, nervousness, confusion, headaches, memory loss). Deficiency also can lead to neurological changes such as numbness and tingling in the hands and feet, tremors and difficulty in maintaining balance. Signs of vitamin B12 deficiency in infancy include: failure to thrive, movement disorders, delayed development, and megaloblastic anemia. One or more of these symptoms does not mean you have B12 deficiency, but you should work with your health care provider to be sure.

So What Can Cause B12 Deficiencies?

Hematologic, neurologic and psychiatric abnormalities, gastricor bowel (ileum surgery, like I've had with my Crohn's disease), folic acid or iron deficiency, prolonged use of stomach acid blockers (proton pump inhibitors, H2 blockers), chronic gastric problems (like I've had), being greater than age 50 (like I am). Some medications may decrease absorption of vitamin B12 (Metformin) and chronic use of those medications may result in a need for additional vitamin B12. Other causes can include: smoking, pregnancy, birth control pills, having a high or low thyroid level, antibiotic use and rarely, being vegan.

Homocysteine

The role of B12 deficiency in hyperhomocysteinemia and the promotion of atherosclerosis is only now being explored. Homocysteine is an amino acid normally found in blood, but elevated levels have been linked with coronary heart disease and stroke. Elevated homocysteine levels may impair endothelial vasomotor function, which determines how easily blood flows through blood vessels. High levels of homocysteine also may damage coronary arteries and make it easier for blood clotting cells called platelets to clump together and form a clot, which may lead to a heart attack Adding folic acid (green leafy veggies) to your diet may help lower homocysteine levels but adding B12 also appears to be essential. Why we need both folic acid and B12 is seen in B12 deficiency anemia. Folic acid can correct the anemia that is caused by vitamin B12 deficiency. Unfortunately, folic acid will not correct the nerve damage also caused by vitamin B12 deficiency. Permanent nerve damage can occur if vitamin B12 deficiency is not treated.

How Do I Know If I Am B12 Deficient?

The diagnosis of vitamin B12 deficiency is typically based on blood measurement of your serum vitamin B12 level; however, about 50 percent of patients with subclinical disease have normal B12 levels. A B12 level in the normal range does not ensure that your B12 levels are healthy. A more sensitive method of screening for vitamin B12 deficiency is measurement of serum methylmalonic acid andhomocysteine levels, which are increased early in vitamin B12 deficiency.

Pernicious Anemia

Anemia can result from a variety of medical problems, including deficiencies of vitamin B12, vitamin B6 folate and iron. But the most famous B12 deficiency is pernicious anemia. It is the name given more than a century ago to describe the then fatal vitamin B12 deficiency anemia that results from severe gastric atrophy, a condition that prevents gastric cells from secreting Intrinsic Factor (IF). IF is a substance normally present in the stomach. Vitamin B12 must bind with IF before it can be absorbed and used by your body. An absence of IF prevents normal absorption of vitamin B12 and results in pernicious anemia. Up to 30 percent of adults aged 50 years and older may have atrophic gastritis and an increased growth of intestinal bacteria, and are unable to normally absorb vitamin B12 from their food. Occasionally, the liver doesn't convert cyanocobalamin into adequate amounts of methylcobalamin. The interruption of one or any combination of these steps places a person at risk of developing B12 deficiency. Our liver stores B12 for between four to twenty years, so it may take years for any symptoms to show up.

What They Didn't Know To Tell Me In Medical School-1970's

When I was in medical training in the late 1970's we used the Schilling test for detection of pernicious anemia (B12 deficiency-lack of functioning IF). Now we use serologic (blood) testing for parietal cell and intrinsic factor antibodies. Low vitamin B12 concentrations in your cells could be the result of a low vitamin B12 intake or due to a disturbance in the absorption, transport or cellular uptake of this vitamin. Vitamin B12 is bound to the protein in food. Hydrochloric acid in the stomach releases vitamin B12 from proteins in foods during digestion and then it is bound to haptocorrin (HC)*. HC is transferred to the duodenum (the first part of the small bowel after the stomach) where IF arrives from the stomach and binds to vitamin B12. The IF-vitamin B12 complex is absorbed via the IF-B12 receptor, and vitamin B12 is subsequently bound to transcobalamin II (TC II) and released into the circulation. TC II facilitates the transport of vitamin B12 in blood to various tissues. Only 20% of the vitamin B12 in plasma is bound to TC II; the remaining 80% is bound to HC (TC 1+TC III).

Why Don't All Vegans Get B12 Deficiency?

Did God make a mistake? "Oops, I forgot to make a supply of B12 for mankind after sin?" Vegans have normal B12 levels, but can't produce B12; but every human, chicken, cow or any other animal can't produce it either. So how do vegetarian humans and animals get their B12? Bacteria in the small bowel manufacture B12 in very small doses. That's why taking antibiotics may cause B12 deficiency, if your other mechanisms of absorption aren't working properly. Mammals need less B12 on a low plant based protein diet, but need more on a high animal based protein diet. More B12 is needed on a low fat diet as well.

There Is A Second Way To Absorb B12

Approximately 1 percent of any oral or bacteria produced B12 is absorbed by TC I-III's second mechanism. This pathway is important in relation to preventing B12 deficiencies, because it bypasses the IF pathway. Once absorbed, vitamin B12 binds to TC II and is transported throughout the body.

Alzheimer's And B12

Researchers have long been interested in the potential connection between vitamin B12 deficiency and dementia. B12 is one of the battery of tests routinely done on new psychiatric patients in the hospital. A recent review examined correlations between cognitive skills, homocysteine levels, and blood levels of folic acid, vitamin B12 and vitamin B6. The authors found that vitamin B12 deficiency may decrease levels of substances needed for the metabolism of neurotransmitters. Neurotransmitters are chemicals that transmit nerve signals. Reduced levels of neurotransmitters may result in neurologic and cognitive impairment. This is why so many of my patients tell me they feel better and think sharper after a B12 shot. It is improving their neurotransmitter function, even with a normal B12 blood level!

Stomach Acid Blockers Block B12 Absorption

Proton pump inhibitors (PPIs) are used to treat gastro esophageal reflux disease (GERD) and peptic ulcer disease. Examples of PPIs are Omeprazole (Prilosec-OTC) and Prevacid, Aciphex, Protonix, Nexium. H2 receptor antagonists are used to treat peptic ulcer disease. Examples are Tagamet, Pepcid AC, Axid and Zantac. PPIs and H2 medications can interfere with vitamin B12 absorption from food by slowing the release of hydrochloric acid into the stomach. This is a concern because acid is needed to release vitamin B12 from food prior to absorption.

Metformin And B12 Deficiency

Metformin (Glucophage, Glumetza, Fortamet, or any diabetic medicine that has 'Met' in its name) normalizes glucose absorption and is a drug used to treat diabetes. Metformin may interfere with calcium metabolism. This may indirectly reduce vitamin B12 absorption because vitamin B12 absorption requires calcium. Surveys suggest that from 10% to 30% of patients taking Metformin have shown evidence of reduced vitamin B12 absorption. In a study involving 21 subjects with type 2 diabetes, researchers found that 17 who were prescribed Metformin experienced a decrease in vitamin B12 absorption. Researchers also found that using calcium carbonate supplements (1,200 mg/day) helped limit the effect of Metformin on vitamin B12 absorption in these individuals.

So What Can I Do?

The route of administration of vitamin B12, to void the IF pathway, can be nasally, under the tongue or under the skin via a shot. Initial recommended dosages for the shot route include 1,000 to 2,000 mcg per day for one week then 1,000 mcg per month for life. Nasal or under the tongue routes include 1,000 to 5000 mcg every day or every other day for one to two weeks, followed by 1000 to 5,000 mcg every one to three months for individuals with B12 deficiency syndrome. Taking high dose B12 by mouth will not usually replace depleted B12 levels because of your faulty mechanism of absorption that caused you to be deficient in the first place.

*HC is also known as transcobalamin I (TC I) and transcobalamin III (TC III).

References:

Bernard MA, Nakonezny PA, Kashner TM. *"The Effect Of Vitamin B12 Deficiency On Older Veterans And Its Relationship To Health,"* J Am Geriatr Soc 1998;46:1199-206. PubMed abstract

Pennypacker LC, Allen RH, Kelly JP, Matthews LM, Grigsby J, Kaye K, et al. *"High Prevalence Of Cobalamin Deficiency In Elderly Outpatients,"* J Am Geriatr Soc 1992;40:1197-204.

Albert MJ. *"Vitamin B12 Synthesis By Human Small Intestine Bacteria,"* Nature, 1980;283:781.

Wasserman IR. *"Intestinal Absorption Of Vitamin B12,"* Lancet, 1960; 1:173-174.

Bradford GS and Taylor CT. *"Omeprazole And Vitamin B12 Deficiency,"* Annals of Pharmacotherapy 1999;33:641-3

Howden CW. *"Vitamin B12 Levels During Prolonged Treatment With Proton Pump Inhibitors,"* J Clin Gastroenterol 2000;30:29-33.

Bauman WA, Shaw S, Jayatilleke K, Spungen AM, Herbert V. *"Increased Intake Of Calcium Reverses The B12 Malabsorption Induced By Metformin,"* Diabetes Care 2000; 23:1227-31.

McKay DL, Perrone G, Rasmussen H, Dallal G, Blumberg JB. *"Multivitamin/Mineral Supplementation Improves Plasma B-Vitamin Status and Homocysteine Concentration In Healthy Older Adults Consuming A Folate-Fortified Diet,"* Journal of Nutrition 2000; 130:3090-6. http://dietarysupplements.info.nih.gov/factsheets/vitamin B12.asp

Lindenbaum J, Healton EB, Savage DG, Brust JC, Garrett TJ, Podell ER, et al. *"Neuropsychiatric Disorders Caused By Cobalamin Deficiency InThe Absence Of Anemia Or Macrocytosis,"* N Engl J Med 1988; 318:1720-8.

Nygard O, Nordrehaug JE, Refsum H, Ueland PM, Farstad M, Vollset SE. *"Plasma Homocysteine Levels And Mortality In Patients With Coronary Artery Disease,"* N Engl J Med 1997;337:230-6.

Lee GR. *"Pernicious Anemia And Other Causes Of Vitamin B12 (cobalamin) Deficiency,"* In: Lee GR, et al., eds. Wintrobe's Clinical hematology. 10th ed. Baltimore: Williams & Wilkins, 1999:941-64.

VITAMIN D

- A Hormone For All People
- The Silent Epidemic

The Sunshine Vitamin

Children are taught in first grade that vitamin D is the "sunshine vitamin." Vitamin D was discovered in 1930 and is both a vitamin and a hormone. It is oil/fat-soluble.* The best source of vitamin D is allowing sunshine to contact your skin. Vitamin D can not be directly produced by our bodies. We humans do not have a requirement for vitamin D when sufficient sunlight is available. Once your body has synthesized enough vitamin D from sunlight exposure, it will produce no more.** "Adults need 10-15 minutes of sunlight (to hands, face and legs), two or three times a week to ensure proper vitamin D levels." Journal of Pediatrics, 1985; 107. Your skin can produce up to 12,000 International Units (IU) of vitamin D in 20 minutes of sunshine.

Why Are We Lacking In Vitamin D?

I haven't seen rickets in 30 years, but most of my patients are deficient in vitamin D. 36% of healthy people and 57% of hospitalized patients had vitamin D deficiency. We have been brain washed to fear skin cancer and wrinkles from sun exposure. We block sunlight by wearing long sleeves and hats, live in cities with tall buildings that block adequate sunlight from reaching the ground, live indoors, use synthetic sun screens that block ultraviolet rays, and live in northern regions of the world that do not receive adequate sunlight, all contributing to the inability of our skin to biosynthesize sufficient amounts of vitamin D_3. The requirement for vitamin D_3 is dependent on our age (older than 60), degree of exposure to the sun, season (winter blood levels drop), obesity (have reduced blood levels) and the amount of pigmentation in our skin (darker skin makes less vitamin D).

What Does Cholesterol Have To Do With Vitamin D?

The basic molecular structure of vitamin D comes from the much maligned hormone cholesterol. Other hormones that use cholesterol as its precursor include: cortisol, estradiol (estrogen), progesterone, aldosterone, and testosterone. All steroid hormones are chemically related to vitamin D_2, D_3 and cholesterol.

The Two Vitamin D's

There are two chemical forms of vitamin D, namely vitamin D_2 (sometimes referred to as ergocalciferol) and vitamin D_3 (sometimes referred to as cholecalciferol). The natural form of vitamin D for mammals (animals and man) is vitamin D3 that is produced in their bodies from cholesterol and 7-dehydrocholesterol. An equally effective alternative is plant based vitamin D2, which is derived from the yeaststerol ergosterol. I was taught in medical school that D3 was superior for supplemental replacement, but vitamin D experts at Boston University (11/07) reported that D2 and D3 were equally effective in maintaining adequate vitamin D levels. Harvard Health Letter, 4/08;33(6):8

Where Does Commercial Vitamin D3 Come From?

Observant Jews, Muslims, Seventh-day Adventists and vegetarians never eat pork, or so they think. In the 1940s, milk was supplemented with vitamin D2, which reduced the incidence rate of juvenile rickets by 85% in the United States. Vitamin D2 is manufactured by exposing bacteria and algae to ultraviolet light. D2 imparted a bitter taste to dairy products, and so was replaced by vitamin D3. Commercially available vitamin D3 always is derived from non kosher sources (Leviticus11). The pro-vitamin known as 7-dehydrocholesterol is extracted via solvent from pig, sheep or cow skin, raw fish liver, and pig brains. It is then exposed to ultraviolet light to produce vitamin D3. Most of the time, 7-dehydrocholesterol is extracted from pig skin and sold to dairy processors. Once chemically pure it is impossible to determine the original animal source (sheep lanolin, pig skin, cow skin, etc.) of crystalline 7-dehydrocholesterol. The exact process is patented (thus secret). Other food sources of vitamin D3 include eggs and fatty fish like cod, salmon, halibut, etc.

How Do I Know If There Is Vitamin D3 Added?

The US Food and Drug Administration (FDA) requires a notice on the label that states "400 IU of added vitamin D3". However, it is not required by law to indicate either the manufacturer or the sources of the D3.

The major producers of vitamin D3 used for milk and other food supplementation are the companies F. Hoffman La Roche, Ltd (Switzerland) and BASF (Germany). In the United States, fortification of foods with vitamin D includes milk (both fresh and evaporated), margarine, butter, soy milk, bread, orange juice, cereals, and chocolate mixes. Other dairy products (cheese, yogurt, etc.) are not fortified with vitamin D, unless labeled.

What's So Good About Vitamin D?

Vitamin D3 is essential for life in higher animals. Vitamin D3 is a regulator of calcium. It stimulates the absorption of calcium from food across the intestine. It helps incorporate the absorbed calcium into your bones. Many studies have looked at the potential of vitamin D to reduce the risk of everything from cancer to diabetes. These benefits from vitamin D are linked to high levels; unfortunately, higher than the usual levels seen in North America. Did you know that persistent, nonspecific musculoskeletal pain correlates with a high risk of unrecognized and untreated vitamin D deficiency? *Mayo Clin Proc 2003;78:1463-70.*

Autism

Recently even autism has been blamed on low vitamin D levels. Both the brain and the blood of autistic individuals show evidence of ongoing chronic inflammation and oxidative stress. Autism is more common in children born to mothers who were vitamin D deficient. "Children with vitamin D rickets have several autistic markers that apparently disappear with high dose vitamin D treatment." says Dr. John Cannell. "Autism and vitamin D," Med hypotheses, Oct 4, 2007. Activated vitamin D stimulates neurotrophin release (neurotrophins induce the survival of nerve cells), reduces toxic calcium levels in the brain, and inhibits the production of nitrous oxide (nitrous oxide destroys brain cells). Besides reducing inflammatory cytokines, vitamin D does one more thing: it increases concentrations of glutathione, the brain's master antioxidant.

Cancer

North Easterners have higher rates of cancer than those in the Southwest because of sunshine! These include: colon, breast, prostate, bladder, esophagus, stomach, kidney, pancreas, rectal, uterine, ovary and non-Hodgkin's lymphoma (there are 17 cancers tracked so far). Active vitamin D fights cancer by slowing or stopping unregulated cell growth (by affecting the growth factors and receptors); it increases the death rate of cancer cells and reduces the blood supply to the tumors. Researchers analyzed multiple studies and found that people with the highest level of D had 50% lower risk of colon and breast cancer. *Am J Prevent Med, 3/07; J Steroid Biochem Molecul Biol, 3/07.* An 18 year study found that men with the lowest level of vitamin D had twice the rate of prostate cancer. *PLoS Med, 3/07.* Treating prostate cancer with high levels of vitamin D reduced the prostate specific antigen (PSA) by 50%. The PSA is a measure of the cancer's aggressiveness.

Hypertension And Your Heart

The farther you live from the equator, the greater your risk of having elevated blood pressure (BP). Vitamin D helps regulate the kidney's production of renin, an enzyme that controls the relaxation and constriction of your arteries. Boston University School of Medicine took one group of people and exposed them to UVB radiation in a tanning bed three times a week for three months. Then they took another group and exposed them to UVA radiation which doesn't boost vitamin D levels. The UVB group had a six point drop in their systolic and diastolic blood pressure (top and bottom BP numbers) and a 180% increase in their blood level of vitamin D. The UVA group had no change in BP or vitamin D levels.

The Framingham study found that the lowest levels of vitamin D correlated with the worst vascular disease (including coronary artery disease). Low levels of vitamin D were also correlated with abnormal blood clotting and abnormal heart rhythms (related to the body's supply of calcium and phosphorus).

Osteoporosis

Low levels of vitamin D can cause and worsen osteoporosis-the bone eroding disease that often leads to hip fractures. Your vitamin D status is more important than your calcium intake in maintaining your parathyroid hormone levels. One in six North Americans will have a hip fracture before they die. For the elderly, one in three men and one in five women with hip fractures will die within one year. More than 50% of those being treated for osteoporosis have low blood levels of vitamin D. Wake Forest University School of Medicine found those with the lowest level of vitamin D had the worst balance and strength, thus the highest rate of falls and fractures. *J Geront: Med Sci, 4/07*. By adding 800 IU of vitamin D in nursing home patients over a five month period, falls were reduced by 72% vs. placebo. *J Am Geriatric Soc, 2/07.* By getting more vitamin D, you will increase your muscle strength and stability.

Multiple Sclerosis (MS) And Autoimmune Disorder

MS is a slowly developing autoimmune disease in which the body's immune system attacks the myelin sheaths that surrounds nerve fibers, brain and your spinal cord. The common symptoms include fatigue, poor balance, memory problems and depression. Harvard School of Public Health found that veterans with the highest levels of vitamin D had a 62% lower risk of developing *MS. JAMA 12/20/06*. MS patients with the highest levels of vitamin D had the least disability. *J Neur 5/07*. Why does vitamin D help? Vitamin D stimulates transforming growth factor (TGF beta-1) and interleukin 4 (IL-4) production, which suppresses inflammatory T cell activity. Any autoimmune disorder (there are over 80) will benefit from vitamin D's powerful anti-inflammatory properties including: thyroiditis, Crohn's disease, inflammatory bowel disease, skin (like psoriasis, eczema, and dermatitis), pernicious anemia, lupus, Sjogren syndrome, autism fibromyalgia and rheumatoid arthritis.

Diabetes

Type 1(juvenile) diabetes is caused by the body's immune system attacking the insulin-secreting cells of the pancreas. A study in Finland gave cod-liver oil (rich in vitamin D) to children during their first year of life and found that they were 78% less likely to develop type 1 diabetes. Type 2 diabetes (adult onset) is caused by the body becoming resistant to the effects of insulin or not producing enough insulin. It is seen more often in vitamin D deficienct patients. Vitamin D helps regulate insulin secretion and increases insulin production.

Polycystic Ovarian Syndrome (PCOS)

PCOS results in reproductive and menstrual dysfunction. In normal calcium patients, vitamin D repletion with calcium therapy resulted in normalizing periods and resolution of pain. Abnormal calcium homeostasis, modulated by vitamin D, may be in part responsible for the arrested follicular development seen in PCOS. *Thys-Jacobs, S., "Vitamin D and calcium dysregulation in the polycystic ovarian syndrome,"Steroids, 6/99;64(6):430-5.*

Peripheral Neuropathy

Peripheral neuropathy can be treated by increasing your sun exposure. Vitamin D3 induces nerve growth factor (NGF) production in the skin, which promotes healing of your painful neuropathy. *Fukuoka,M., Skin Pharm Appl Skin Physiol, 7-8/01;14(4):226-33.*

Do I Need To Take Vitamin D?

There is an epidemic in clinically proven hypo-vitaminosis D in all age groups, seen even in Florida. One fourth of all teenagers are vitamin D deficient. Should I consider more sunshine or taking a vitamin D supplement (D2 plant-based source or D3 animal-based source)? Vitamin D toxicity is very rare. Your physician can measure a serum 25-hydroxy-vitamin D level for about $100. Most of my patient need sunshine and 2000 IU/day. Vitamin D can be made by your skin from sunlight through the window, so you can stay inside if it is too hot or cold outside. Just expose as much skin as possible!

* There are two general chemical categories of vitamins based on their solubility: water soluble vitamins (the B and C vitamins) and fat soluble vitamins (A, D, E and K).

** Exposure of our skin to sunlight results in the photochemical conversionof 7-dehydrocholesterol into vitamin D3. This sunlight- generated vitamin D3 is a precursor of the steroid hormone 1,25(OH)2D3 which is activated in our livers and kidneys.

References:

Norman, A.W., *"An Introduction To Vitamin D: With Emphasis on the Topics of Chemistry, Sources, Production, Presence in Milk and Nutritional Importance,"* Department of Biochemistry & Biomedical Sciences, University of California, Riverside CA 92521:2000.

Holick, M., *"High Prevalence of Vitamin D inadequacy and Implications for Health,"* Mayo Clinc Proc, 2006:81(3):353-73.

University Of California, Berkeley, Wellness Letter, *"Vitamin D: are you getting enough?"* Vol24:5; 2/08:1-2.

Harris, S.S. and Dawson-Hughes,B. *"Seasonal changes in plasma 25- hydroxy-vitamin D concentrations of young American black and white women."* Am.J.Clin.Nutr. 67 (1998) 1232-1236.

Adams, J.S., Clemens,T.L., Parrish,J.A., and Holick,M.F. *"Vitamin-D synthesis and metabolism after ultraviolet irradiation of normal and vitamin-D-deficient subjects."* New Engl.J.Med. 306 (1982) 722-725.

Webb, A.R., Pilbeam,C., Hanafin,N., and Holick,M.F. *"An evaluation of the relative contributions of exposure to sunlight and of diet to the circulatingconcentrations of 25-hydroxy-vitamin D in an elderly nursing homepopulation in Boston."* Am.J.Clin.Nutr. 51(6) (1990) 1075-1081. http://www.vitamindcouncil.org/health/autism/

Wicherts, I.S., *"Vitamin D status predicts physical performance and its decline in older persons,"* J Clin Endocrinol Metab, Mar 6, 2007.

Park, S, *"Living in low-latitude regions in the United States dose notprevent poor vitamin D status."* Nutr Rev. June 2005; 63(6pt1):203-9.

HEAVEN'S GIFT OF SUNSHINE

No one wants skin cancer, and no one wants wrinkled aged skin! So - 'stay out of the sun' we are told. We try. We cover up; we put on plenty of sunscreen, or we just stay indoors. But how can anything as wonderful as sunlight be so harmful to our health? Like almost everything in life, too much of a good thing can be a bad thing. But in proper amounts, sunlight is a great blessing. Besides warming our earth and making things grow... sunlight is an efficient germ killer. Proper amounts of sunshine also give the skin a healthy glow and help make it smooth and pliable. In addition, a moderately tanned skin is more resistant to infections and sunburns than untanned skin. Sunlight lifts the spirits of most people, producing a cheerful sense of well-being. Combined with active exercise, sunshine is an important aid in treating acute and chronic depression. In fact, seasonal variations in light levels can have a profound effect on one's mental health. These effects may be clearly seen in people suffering from seasonal affective disorder. This is a depressive illness associated with the small amounts of sunlight in fall and winter. Sunlight is a simple yet very successful treatment for this condition. So during winter's cold and gloomy months, try and catch any possible extra rays of sunshine.

Sunshine also plays a crucial role in helping to prevent osteoporosis. The body is able to manufacture vitamin D by the action of sunlight on the skin. This Vitamin D enables the body to utilize the calcium essential for building healthy bones. A deficiency of Vitamin D leads to rickets, a disorder where children's bones become soft and weak. Did you know that daily sunlight also helps promote better sleep? In recent years, melatonin, a natural body hormone, has been found to enhance sleep. The body carefully regulates melatonin production. The process is largely controlled by the light-dark cycle. Optimal melatonin production occurs at night, in a dark environment, especially after a bright sunny day. Melatonin is not stored in the body. We need a liberal supply each evening to sleep well. Studies demonstrate that daily exposure to natural sunlight will boost melatonin output. Artificial light is a weak substitute, as are manufactured melatonin supplements. Melatonin levels reach a peak in children, and fall slowly and steadily throughout adult life. This may explain why children sleep so much better than older people. In addition to what we've already mentioned, sunlight strengthens the immune system, alleviates pain from swollen arthritic joints, and may lower elevated blood pressure and cholesterol levels. An extra hour of sunlight every day, besides lifting your spirits, may also positively affect your energy, sleep, and even PMS (premenstrual syndrome).

But What About Skin Cancer?

It's true; **overexposure** to sunlight does increase skin cancer risk, especially in light-skinned people. About 95 percent of skin cancers are of two types: **Squamous cell cancer,** and **Basal cell cancer**. The chances of developing these types of cancer are increased when the skin is exposed to liberal doses of sunshine over many years. Fortunately, however, both of these cancers are slow growing and usually remain confined to the skin. There are very few fatalities, and these are mostly in people who neglect to have the cancers promptly removed. Melanoma is a third type of skin cancer, which is very different from the others. It usually begins with a darkly pigmented mole, and has a fearsome tendency to spread and kill the victim. The rates of Melanoma cancer are rapidly rising around the world. The important risk factor with melanoma is sunburn, not so much the total amount of sunlight people are exposed to. Burning the skin is extremely harmful. Every burn destroys healthy, living tissue. Repeated burns cause irreversible damage and can cause skin cancer. And if all that isn't bad enough, repeated sunburn and even repeated deep tanning of the skin gradually destroys its elasticity and its oil glands, producing wrinkling and premature aging. Therefore, overdoses of sunlight should be carefully avoided. Dietary choices can also affect our chances of getting skin cancer. A high-fat diet, so common in today's society, significantly increases a person's risk. On the other hand, a diet with plenty of antioxidant-rich fruits and vegetables can help protect us from many types of cancers. Diets high in vitamin C and E have been shown to offer significant protection against skin cancer in particular. The best way to obtain healthy amounts of theses antioxidant vitamins is to eat the foods that contain them. Vitamin C is found in abundance in fresh vegetables and fruit, such as red and green bell peppers, green leafy vegetables, strawberries, blueberries and all citrus fruits. Some good sources of Vitamin E include almonds and sunflower seeds, green soybeans, sunflower oil, canola oil, olive oil, and even cooked spinach. It's important to emphasize that most of the studies showing the cancer-protective effects of antioxidants have involved people who were getting their vitamins from natural foods, not vitamins from a bottle. Some of the research indicates that vitamin supplements do not provide the same protection that the natural food sources of these vitamins give. Speaking of which, did you know that sunshine could actually help to prevent it?

People who get adequate sunshine are less likely to develop breast, colon or prostate cancer. Researchers have also observed that the vitamin D and related compounds formed as a result of exposure to sunlight appear to suppress the growth of cancers already present. This includes certain types of leukemia and lymphoma, as well as breast and colon cancers. What can you to do to maximize sunlight's benefits, while avoiding the harmful effects of getting too much?

Some Suggestions For Safe, Healthy Exposure To Sunlight

Modest tanning is protective; it's like putting sunglasses on your skin. But each person must understand his or her tolerance to sunlight. Fair-skinned people may need to begin with only five minutes of exposure to the sun per day, with up to 30 minutes of sunbathing as a realistic goal for most people. Remember; NEVER BURN! Sunburns raise the risk of skin cancer. Wear protective clothing, eye-wear, and a protective sunscreen if needed. Be especially careful around snow or water and on cloudy days because of the reflected rays and the ultraviolet rays that penetrate through clouds. If you have an outdoor trip or vacation coming up, prepare your skin by giving it progressive exposure to sunlight in the days beforehand. Get a few minutes of sunshine on your face and hands each day. This will produce all the vitamin D you need for a healthy body and strong bones. Just remember that artificial light is a very poor substitute for the real thing. Spend a little time each day soaking up some daylight. Open your house to the sunshine each morning. It will improve your health and lift your spirits. For thousands of years, sunlight has been known as a mediator of life. Today we know that a wise use of sunlight can be extremely beneficial. It can be either healing or destructive on how we choose to use it. In the beginning, when God created the world, He said," Let there be light," and there was light. And God saw that the light, that it was good." Genesis 1: 3, 4. May God bless you as you seek to make a wise use of sunlight- one of heaven's nicest gifts.

Health talk given by Jillionna Bailey 7/12/06, age 15.

APPLE FACTS

- The crab apple is the only apple native to North America.
- Two pounds of apples make one 9-inch pie.
- Apple blossom is the state flower of Michigan.
- 2,500 varieties of apples are grown in the United States. 7,500 varieties of apples are grown throughout the world. 100 varieties of apples are grown commercially in the United States. Apples are grown commercially in 36 states. Apples are grown in all 50 states. Apples come in all shades of reds, greens, and yellows. In 2005, there were7500 apple growers with orchards covering 379,000 acres.
- North Carolina has over 200 commercial apple operations comprised of 9,000 bearing acres of apple orchards. Up to 4 million bushels of apples can be produced in North Carolina in a given year. Apples are produced in four areas of the state around the Henderson, Haywood, Wilkes and Cleveland areas. The four major varieties which make up the bulk of NC's production are Red Delicious, Golden Delicious, Rome Beauty and Galas.
- A medium apple is about 80 calories. Don't peel your apple. Two-thirds of the fiber and lots of antioxidants are found in the peel. Apples are rich in fiber pectin. Pectin and mild acids found in apples help fight body toxins, aid digestion and pep up the whole system. Pectin, too has been associated with helping to keep cholesterol levels in balance. Flavonoids in apples play a role in prevention of certain cancers and heart disease. One apple has five grams of fiber. The high potassium/low sodium ratio is important in certain cardiac and renal problems as well as in diets for overweight persons. Studies have shown that persons eating apples regularly have fewer headaches and other illnesses associated

with nervous tension. Other studies have demonstrated an association of regular apple consumption with a reduced incidence of colds and other upper respiratory ailments. Apples are "Nature's Toothbrush." The mild fibrous texture of the apple, its non-adherent nature, juice content and mouth watering appeal to accelerate salivary action all combine to make it a wonderful natural aid for cleansing teeth. Apples contain zero fat per serving and no cholesterol or trans fats.

- Always refrigerate your apples as cold as possible without freezing. Apples will ripen and therefore turn soft 10 times faster at room temperature, and nearly 5 times faster at 40 degrees F.
- Apples stored in commercial refrigerated storage will keep for 4-6months, but can be stored long term up to 12 months. The apples are rushed into storage the day they are picked. The oxygen level is lowered to 1.5-3%, temperature is reduced to 30-32 F, and carbon dioxide levels are monitored and controlled.
- The pilgrims planted the first United States apple trees in the Massachusetts Bay Colony.
- The science of apple growing is called pomology.
- Apple trees take four to five years to produce their first fruit.
- Peak harvest of NC hand picked apples is mid August through October.
- Apple varieties range in size from a little larger than a cherry to as large as a grapefruit.
- Apples are propagated by two methods: grafting or budding.
- Apples were the favorite fruit of ancient Greeks and Romans.
- Apples are a member of the rose family.
- Apples harvested from an average tree can fill 20 boxes that weigh 42 pounds each.
- A bushel of apples weights about 42 pounds and will yield 20-24 quarts of applesauce.
- The largest apple picked weighed three pounds.
- The average size of a United States orchard is 50 acres. Many growers use dwarf apple trees.
- Most apple blossoms are pink when they open but gradually fade to white.
- Some apple trees will grow over 40 feet high and live over 100 years.
- Most apples can be grown farther north than most other fruits, because they blossom late in spring, minimizing frost damage.

• It takes the energy from 50 leaves to produce one apple.

• Apples are the second most valuable fruit grown in the United States. Oranges are first.

• In colonial times, apples were called winter banana or melt-in-the-mouth.

• Apples have five seed pockets or carpels. Each pocket contains seeds. The number of seeds per carpel is determined by the vigor and health of the plant. Different varieties of apples will have different number of seeds.

• World's top apple producers are China, United States, Turkey, Poland and Italy.

• The Lady or Api apple is one of the oldest varieties in existence.

• Newton Pippin apples were the first apples exported from America in 1768. Some were sent to Benjamin Franklin in London.

• In 1730 the first apple nursery was opened in Flushing, New York.

• One of George Washington's hobbies was pruning his apple trees.

• America's longest-lived apple tree was reportedly planted in 1647 by Peter Stuyvesant in his Manhattan orchard and was still bearing fruit when a derailed train struck it in 1866.

• A peck of apples weighs 10.5 pounds.

• The world's largest apple peel was created by Kathy Wafler Madison on October 16, 1976, in Rochester, NY. It was 172 feet, 4 inches long. (She was 16 years old at the time and grew up to be a sales manager for an apple tree nursery.)

• It takes about 36 apples to create one gallon of apple cider.

• Apples account for 50 percent of the world's deciduous fruit tree production.

• What makes apples turn red? The cool nights of late August and early September trigger the change in the enzymes of the apple skin to change the color from green to red. This same condition will put a pink "blush" on green Granny Smiths and add the yellow color to Golden Delicious Apples.

• The old saying "An apple a day, keeps the doctor away" comes from an old English adage, "To eat an apple before going to bed, will make the doctor beg his bread."

• In 2005, United States consumers ate an average of 46.1 pounds of fresh apples and processed apple products. That's a lot of applesauce!

- In 2005, 36 percent of apples were processed into apple products; 18.6 percent of this was for juice and cider, two percent was dried, 2.5 percent was frozen, 12.2 percent was canned and 0.7 percent was fresh slices. Other uses were the making of baby food, apple butter or jelly and vinegar.
- In 2006, 58% of apples produced in the United States were produced in Washington, 11% in New York, 8% in Michigan, 5% in Pennsylvania, 4% in California, 2% in Virginia, 2% North Carolina.
- Total apple production in the United States in 2005 was 234.9 million cartons valued at $1.9 billion.
- In 2006/2007 the People's Republic of China led the world in commercial apple production with 24,480,000 metric tons followed by the United States with 4,460,544 metric tons.
- In 2006/2007 commercial world production of apples was 44,119,244 metric tons.
- Almost one out of every four apples harvested in the United States is exported.
- 35.7 million bushels of fresh market apples in 2005 were exported. That was 24 percent of the total U.S. fresh-market crop.
- The apple variety 'Red Delicious' is the most widely grown in the United States with 62 million bushels harvested in 2005.
- Many apples after harvesting and cleaning have commercial grade wax applied. Waxes are made from natural ingredients.
- On August 21, 2007 the GoldRush apple was designated as the official Illinois state fruit. GoldRush is a sweet-tart yellow apple with a long shelf life. The apple is also the state fruit of Minnesota, New York, Vermont, Washington and West Virginia.

Apple Nutrition Facts

(*One medium 2 1/2 inch apple, fresh, raw, with skin)

Calories 81

Carbohydrates 21 grams
Dietary Fiber 4 grams
Soluble Fiber
Insoluble fiber
Calcium 10 mg
Phosphorus 10 mg
Iron .25 mg
Sodium 0.00 mg
Potassium 159 mg
Vitamin C 8 mg
Vitamin A 73 IU
Folate 4 mcg

Keep Your Mind Sharp • Eat An Apple

BERRY GOOD

"Our data indicate for the first time that it may be possible to overcome genetic predisposition to Alzheimer's disease through diet."
-Nutritional Science, Apr. 2004

New Studies

New research indicates that in animal studies regular consumption of blueberries can prevent age-related memory problems. Similar antioxidant-rich findings are associated with raspberries, blackberries, cranberries and strawberries, etc. Blueberry (BB) supplementation reversed the deleterious effects of aging on motor behavior and neuronal signaling with no alterations in amyloid beta burden. Amyloid deposits in the human brain have been correlated with advancing memory deterioration. Protective mechanisms are derived from BB-induced enhancement of memory.*

Nuclear Factor Kappa B (NF-kB)

NF-kB is a rapid oxidative (rusting out process) stress response protein. It is a transcription factor in all cells involved in immune and inflammatory reactions. NF-kB exerts its effects by expressing cytokines, chemokines, cell adhesion molecules, growth factors and immunoreceptors. Hyper proliferating cells (like in cancer) often over-express NF-kB and use this as a growth vehicle to escape cell regulatory control. NF-kB contributes to autoimmune disorders (like my Crohn's Disease or Lupus, Parkinsonism, Thyroiditis, Alzheimer's, Colitis, and even Psoriasis, to name a few). NF-kB contributes to allograft rejection (failure of transplanted organs, like kidneys, hearts, livers, etc), rheumatoid arthritis and bronchial asthma.

Blue Berries And Memory

So why have I told you about NF-kB? Because 2% BB supplementation prevented elevated levels of NF-kB, thus preventing or slowing the progression of an autoimmune disease. BB supplementation prevented impaired object recognition memory by normalizing or lowering NF-kB levels. Therefore, the use of BBs correlated significantly with improved object memory scores.

Pterostilbene

Blueberries contain the highest level of folic acid in any fruit. They also contain pterostilbene. Pterostilbene's properties are similar to the compound resveratrol, found in purple grapes and are the chemical that gives the health benefit in red wine. Pterostilbene has strong antioxidant capabilities, is a potent cancer-preventive agent, and has been shown to help protect the heart and cardiovascular system. Pterostilbene lowers glucose levels in animals by 42% without any side effects. Pterostilbene inhibits platelets aggregation and increases the good (Happy) HDL form of cholesterol. Pterostilbene is also found in darker grapes, but not in red wine (it doesn't survive the wine-making process). It is the pterostilbene in BB (and other berries) that is believed to be the memory enhancing antioxidant.

So, start adding those berries, fresh, dried, or frozen to your diet.

*Through memory associated neuronal signaling (extracellular signal-regulated kinase) and alterations in neutral sphingomyelin-specific phospholipase C activity.

References:

Goyarzu,P., *"Blueberry Supplemented Diet: Effects On Object Recognition Memory And Nuclear Factor-kappa B Levels In Aged Rats,"* Nutritional Neuroscience, April 2004; vol.7, no.2:75-83.

Joseph, J.A., *"Blueberry Supplementation Enhances Signaling And Prevents Behavioral Deficits in an Alzheimer Disease Model,"* Nutritional Neuroscience, May 2003; vol.6, no.3:153-162.

Williams,D., *"A Berry Good Solution,"* Alternatives, November 2004:134.

Lee,J.L., *"Nuclear Factor Kappa B: Important Transcription Factor And Therapeutic Target,"* J Clin Phar, 1998;38:981-993.

CELERY

- The Healthy Vegetable

Celery became popular first as a medicine and then later as a food. Celery was found in King Tut's tomb. Celery is mentioned in Homer's Odyssey. Celery is a crunchy vegetable that belongs to the Apiaceae family; the same plant family as carrots, parsley, fennel and caraway. Celery has 6 calories per eight inch stalk (one cup = 19 calories).

Celery contains per cup-chopped: Calcium 48 mg, folate 33.6, iron .48 mg, magnesium 13.2 mg, tryptophan .01 grams, manganese .12 mg, phosphorous 30 mg, potassium 344 mg, vitamin A 160.8 IU, vitamin B1 .06 mg, vitamin B2 .05 mg, vitamin B6 .10 mg, vitamin C 8.4 mg, vitamin K 35.26 mcg, molybdenum 6 mcg. Other contents of celery include: amino acids, boron, essential fatty acids, inositol, selenium, zinc, vitamin E, Vitamin B3 and vitamin B5. Celery is also high in fiber (2 grams of fiber/cup). It cleans your teeth and keeps your gums healthy. When wrapped in aluminum foil, the stalk will stay fresh for several weeks in the refrigerator.

The health benefits of celery include:

Reduced blood pressure: Celery contains a chemical (phthalides) that can lower levels of stress hormones in your blood. This allows blood vessels to expand, giving your blood more room, thereby reducing your overall pressure. Celery is known as a high sodium food but it is not. One cup = 100 mg of sodium (Sodium allowance is 2400 mg/day). Blend for 10 ounces and drink twice a day minimum.

Reduced cholesterol: Eating celery daily increases your bile acid production, which will reduce your artery-clogging cholesterol level. Cholesterol is in the bile and the more you eat, the lower your cholesterol will go.

Weight loss: Celery is high in fiber; eating one to two stalks before meals fills you up and decreases the volume of food you consume. Drinking celery juice before meals will help you to reduce your weight also.

Good antiseptic: Celery seeds help in uric acid elimination. So, celery is good for people with bladder disorders, kidney problems and cystitis. Celery seeds also assist in avoiding urinary tract infection in women.

Constipation: Celery increases bile acids in your small bowels, which loosen your stools as well as adds fiber to eliminate constipation. Start with one stalk three times a day.

Healthy joints: Celery is good for people suffering from arthritis, rheumatism and gout. Its anti-inflammatory properties help reduce swelling and pain around the joints. Celery sticks contain a diuretic substance, which help to remove uric acid crystals that build around joints.

Prevents cancer: Celery contains phthalides and polyacetylenes. These anti cancer components detoxify carcinogens and have been shown to stop the growth of tumor cells. Celery contains compounds called coumarins that help prevent free radicals from damaging your cells, thus decreasing the mutations that increase the potential for cells to become cancer. Coumarins also enhance the activity of certain white blood cells, immune defenders that target and eliminate potentially harmful cells, including cancer cells. Celery helps alkalize your body from chronic acid loads we encounter in our environment and foods. Start with one stalk three times a day working up to drinking blended celery 10 ounces, minimum twice daily.

Improved immune system: Celery is rich in vitamin C and will raise your body Ph to help boost your immune system.

Relief from colds: Because of the presence of vitamin C and its alkaline base, eating celery can give you relief from flu symptoms.

Reduces severity of asthma: Vitamin C prevents free radical damage, and thus reduces the severity of inflammatory conditions like asthma.

Cardiovascular health: Presence of vitamin C in the roots of celery promotes cardiovascular health. Celery also acts as an antioxidant.

Diuretic activity: Celery is rich in both natural sodium and potassium. These minerals help in regulating fluid balance, thus stimulating urine flow.

Relief from migraine: Presence of coumarins gives relief from migraines. Take two 10 ounce glasses of blended celery a day.

Good for diabetic patients: Celery leaves are also eaten around the world for treating diabetic conditions.

Relief from ophthalmologic disease: Dripping celery tea drops on eyelids is good for ophthalmologic affectations.

Calms the nerves: Because of celery's high calcium content and tryptophan, celery calms your nerves.

All parts of the celery including the seeds, root and leaves, can be eaten. I have found celery stalks very soothing to my Crohn's diseased gut. During my flares, celery is one of the only foods that doesn't upset my bowels. I like it raw, in salads, soups, casseroles and with peanut and nut butters on it.

References:
http://www.whfoods.com/genpage.php?tname=foodspice&dbid=14
http://www.organicfacts.net/health-benefits/vegetable/health-benefits-of-celery.html

THE AMAZING CUCUMBER

- I'm Putting Cucumbers On My Grocery List Today!!

Maybe We Should All Try This??

Note: This information was in The New York Times, internet dated 11-17-09, as part of their "Spotlight on the Home" series that highlighted creative and fanciful ways to solve common problems.

1. Cucumbers contain most of the vitamins you need every day. Just one cucumber contains Vitamin B1, Vitamin B2, Vitamin B3, Vitamin B5, Vitamin B6, Folic Acid, Vitamin C, Calcium, Iron, Magnesium, Phosphorus, Potassium and Zinc.

2. Feeling tired in the afternoon? Put down the caffeinated soda and pick up a cucumber! Cucumbers are a good source of B Vitamins and Carbohydrates that can provide a quick pick-me-up that can last for hours.

3. Tired of your bathroom mirror fogging up after a shower? Try rubbing a cucumber slice along the mirror; it will eliminate the fog and provide a soothing, spa-like fragrance.

4. Are grubs and slugs ruining your planting beds? Place a few slices in a small pie tin and your garden will be free of pests all season long. The chemicals in the cucumber react with the aluminum to give off a scent undetectable to humans but that drives garden pests crazy and makes them flee the area.

5. Looking for a fast and easy way to remove cellulite before going out or to the pool? Try rubbing a slice or two of cucumbers along your problem area for a few minutes. The phytochemicals in the cucumber cause the collagen in your skin to tighten, firming up the outer layer and reducing the visibility of cellulite. Works great on wrinkles too!!!

6. Want to avoid that migraine or terrible headache? Eat a few cucumber slices before going to bed and wake up refreshed and headache free. Cucumbers contain enough sugar, B vitamins and electrolytes to replenish essential nutrients the body lost, keeping everything in equilibrium, avoiding your headache!!

7. Looking to fight off that afternoon or evening snacking binge? Cucumbers have been used for centuries and often used by European trappers, traders and explorers for quick meals to thwart off starvation.

8. Have an important meeting or job interview and you realize that you don't have enough time to polish your shoes? Rub a freshly cut cucumber over the shoe. Its chemicals will provide a quick and durable shine that not only looks great but also repels water.

9. Out of WD-40, and need to fix a squeaky hinge? Take a cucumber slice and rub it along the problematic hinge, and voila, the squeak is gone!

10. Stressed out and don't have time for massage, facial or visit to the spa? Cut up an entire cucumber and place it in a boiling pot of water. The chemicals and nutrients from the cucumber react with the boiling water and are released in the steam, creating a soothing, relaxing aroma that has been shown to reduce stress in new mothers and college students during final exams.

11. Just finish a business lunch and realize you don't have gum or mints? Take a slice of cucumber and press it to the roof of your mouth with your tongue for 30 seconds to eliminate bad breath. The phytochemcials will kill the bacteria in your mouth responsible for causing bad breath.

12. Looking for a 'green' way to clean your faucets, sinks or stainless steel? Take a slice of cucumber and rub it on the surface you want to clean. Not only will it remove years of tarnish and bring back the shine, but it won't leave streaks and won't harm your fingers or fingernails while you clean.

13. Using a pen and made a mistake? Take the outside of the cucumber and slowly use it to erase the pen writing. This also works great on crayons and markers that the kids have used to decorate your walls!!

BELL PEPPERS

- Super Food

Bell peppers (sweet peppers) are from the species Capsicum annuum- the chili pepper family. They contain a recessive gene that eliminates capsaicin, the compound responsible for the 'hotness' found in other peppers. The bell pepper is one of the vegetables in the nightshade *(Solanaceae)* family, which include eggplant, tomatoes and white potatoes. They get their name because they are shaped like a bell.

Origin

Bell peppers are native to Mexico, Central America and northern South America. Pepper seeds were carried by Columbus to Spain in 1493 and from there spread to other European, African and Asian countries. Today, Mexico remains one of the major pepper producers in the world.

Antioxidants Vitamin C And A

Peppers are excellent sources of vitamin C (175 mg/cup) and vitamin A (5244 iu per cup), two very powerful antioxidants. These antioxidants work together to effectively neutralize free radicals, which can travel through the body causing tremendous amounts of damage to our cells. Free radicals are responsible for: the build up of cholesterol in your arteries that leads to atherosclerosis and heart disease, the nerve and blood vessel damage seen in diabetes, the cloudy lenses of cataracts, the joint pain and damage seen in osteoarthritis and rheumatoid arthritis, and the wheezing and airway tightening of asthma. By consuming these two potent free radical destroyers, bell peppers may help prevent or reduce some of the symptoms of these conditions by shutting down the free radical source of the problem.

Vitamin B6 And Folic Acid For Reducing Homocysteine

For hardening of the arteries and diabetic heart disease, peppers also contain vitamin B6 (0.23 mg per cup) and folic acid (24 mcg per cup). These two B vitamins are very important for reducing high levels of homocysteine, a substance produced during the methylation cycle (an essential biochemical process in virtually every cell in the body). High homocysteine levels have been shown to cause damage to blood vessels and are associated with a greatly increased risk of heart attack and stroke. In addition to providing the vitamins that convert homocysteine into other beneficial molecules, bell peppers also provide fiber (1.84 grams per cup) that can help lower high cholesterol levels, another risk factor for heart attack and stroke.

Less Cancer When You Eat Lycopene-Rich Foods

Red peppers contain lycopene, a carotenoid that correlates with the more you eat the less likely you will get prostate cancer and cancers of the cervix, bladder and pancreas. Recent studies suggest that individuals whose diets are low in lycopene-rich foods are at greater risk for developing these types of cancers.

Colon Cancer

The plant fiber found in peppers can help to reduce the amount of contact that colon cells have with cancer-causing toxins found in certain foods or produced by certain gut bacteria. In addition, consumption of vitamin C, beta-carotene, and folic acid, all found in bell peppers, is associated with a significantly reduced risk of colon cancer.

Reduced Lung Cancer Risk

Consuming foods rich in beta-cryptoxanthin, an orange-red carotenoid found in highest amounts in red bell peppers, pumpkin, corn, papaya, tangerines, oranges and peaches, may significantly lower one's risk of developing lung cancer. If you or someone around you is a smoker, or if you are frequently exposed to secondhand smoke, then making vitamin A-rich foods, such as bell peppers, part of your healthy way of eating may save your life.

Protects You From Eye Damage

Bell peppers have a protective effect against cataracts, due to their vitamin C and beta-carotene content. Italian researchers compared the diets of hospital patients who had cataracts removed with patients who had not undergone the operation. Certain vegetables, including sweet peppers, reduced the cataract operation risk. The red variety of bell peppers also supplies the phytonutrients lutein and zeaxanthin, which have been found to protect against macular degeneration, the main cause of blindness in the elderly.

Arthritis

While one study suggests that high doses of supplemental vitamin C makes osteoarthritis, a type of degenerative arthritis that occurs with aging, worse in laboratory animals, another indicates that vitamin C-rich foods, such as bell and chili peppers, provide humans with protection against inflammatory polyarthritis, a form of rheumatoid arthritis involving two or more joints.

What Color Is Best?

Green bell peppers are the most plentiful year-round. They are also the least expensive, as harvesting is done before ripening. This allows time during the growing season for multiple crops. Green bells are high in folic acid and are slightly bitter by comparison to ripened peppers. Yellow and orange bells are the color phases of the semi-ripened pepper. They are more expensive than green bells and sweeter. Yellow bell peppers are usually juicier than reds. Red bells are, along with yellows, the most expensive and have higher concentrations of Vitamin C. Reds have reached the final ripening stage. Prices will drop in the fall after harvesting, but the plants produce only one crop throughout each season. Hybrids vary in size and shape as well as colors, which include white, purple, brown, and almost black. Attractive in salads; some will turn green when cooked.

Quick Serving Ideas

The Bailey family eats bell peppers every day.

- Add chopped bell peppers (multiple colors) to your salads.
- Steam cored bell peppers for five minutes; stuff them with your favorite rice salad or grain pilaf, and bake in a 350° F oven until they are hot.
- Sauté chopped bell peppers, celery and onions then combine with tofu to make a simple Louisiana Creole dish. I add garlic too.
- Purée roasted and peeled bell peppers with sautéed onions and zucchini to make a deliciously refreshing soup that can be served hot or cold.
- Bell peppers are one of the best vegetables to serve in a veggie platter since not only do they add brilliant color, but their texture is also the perfect crunchy complement for dips.

References:
http://www.whfoods.com/genpage.php?tname=foodspice&dbid=50
http://en.wikipedia.org/wiki/Bell_pepper
http://www.bigoven.com/glossary/Bell%20Pepper

RED FRUIT

- Tastes Great
- Protects From Disease

Red fruit can be a powerful guardian for your health. Red fruits are loaded with beneficial plant compounds called phytochemicals. They preserve your health by keeping your brain agile as you age, guard against heart disease and cancer, ease arthritis, and ward off urinary tract infections and stomach ulcers. Many phytochemicals are antioxidants, which fight off health-damaging free radicals. Here are five of my favorites:

Watermelon - *fights cancer*

Watermelons are 92% water, but help fight off disease by their nutrients: vitamin C, A and potassium. Watermelon contains an amino acid called citrulline that has a diuretic effect, good for those with water retention. You knew that though, didn't you? Did you know that watermelon has 60% more antioxidant lycopene than tomatoes? Studies suggest that lycopene can prevent cancer-cell growth and keeps existing cancer cells from spreading, particularly breast, colon and prostate.

Red Berries - *helps your memory*

Strawberries and raspberries are members of the rose family. They share two important phytochemicals: anthocyanins and ellagic acid. Anthocyanins in berries protect your brain from age-related decline. Ellagic acid in berries helps fight cancer in two ways: by protecting normal cells from damage, and by helping cancer cells die.

Red Grapefruit - *lowers your cholesterol*

Everybody knows that grapefruit has a lot of vitamin C, but they also contain pectin, a soluble fiber that can lower cholesterol. Pectin can also hold cancer cells in check. Another benefit is D-glucaric acid which can lower LDL cholesterol. Grapefruit has more D-glucaric acid than any other fruit or vegetable. Grapefruit has a good amount of glutathione, an amino acid compound the enhances Vitamin C and boosts cell immunity. They also contain naringin, an antioxidant flavonoid that has been shown to reduce atherosclerosis (hardening of the arteries). Why red grapefruit over other colors? Because of the red grapefruit's anti-oxidant pigment beta carotene and lycopene. The redder the more cancer-protective effects they contain.

Cranberries - *helps prevent infections*

These tiny tart phytochemical rich fruits contain more antioxidant phenols than any other fruit. Phenols belong to a group of compounds similar to red grapes, which have been studied for their heart-protective benefits. Phenols reduce total cholesterol and LDL (bad) cholesterol. Cranberries are famous for their ability to ward off urinary tract infections via their tannins, which prevent bacteria from sticking to the walls of the bladder. Ten ounces a day of at least 27% cranberry juice gives you the maximum benefit of phenols and tannins. Cranberries also have compounds that prevent dental plaque and the bacteria Heliobactor pylori (which can cause non-healing stomach ulcers).

Cherries - *can ease your pain*

Ripe, juicy cherries have been found to contain at least 17 antioxidant compounds. Tart and sweet cherries have the same compounds in them, but tart cherries contain more of them. Just 35 tart cherries can reduce pain and inflammation better than aspirin. The reason is they too contain anthocyanins, which inhibit inflammation. They have been used for centuries to treat gout. Cherries are a great source of melatonin, a hormone that your body uses to regulate its sleep patterns and that has been shown to help in irritable bowel problems. They are rich in quercetin, a flavonoid that has been shown to have anti-cancer and anti-oxidant powers. Cherries also contain perillyl alcohol, which has been found to inhibit breast, ovarian and prostate cancers.

References:
Redmond,C., "Reap The Goodness Of Red Fruit," HYPERLINK "http://www.naturalhealthmag.com;" www.naturalhealthmag.com; May/June 2002:66-69.

THE RICE STUFF

Wheat Or Gluten Gensitive? Try Sprouting The Grain!

Rice

If you're making a rice dish, soak the whole brown rice first. According to a Japanese study, soaking brown rice in warm water (crock pot at 90° F) over 22 hours before cooking it can more than double its nutritional value. "As rice soaks, it releases enzymes that not only increases its fiber, vitamin and mineral content, but also boost antioxidant and amino acid levels," says Hiroshi Kayahara, PhD, the study author. Soaking rice also makes it taste sweeter, since the germination that triggers the release of the enzymes also brings out (breaks down) the sugar and protein flavors within the grain. White rice will not germinate because it has been stripped of its outer layers causing this process not to occur.

Sprouted Grains Are More Alkaline

Sprouted seeds, rice and grains become more alkaline in the process of sprouting. Changing its from an acid, pre soaked, to an alkaline food source, post soaked. Alkaline foods help your body use less energy in its never ending battle to maintain your acid-base (Ph) balance. A healthy diet is predominately alkaline in effect (fruits, millet, buckwheat, rice, lentils, soy and lima beans), while an unhealthy diet is predominately acid in effect (sugar, eggs, meats, breads and nuts, except almonds and brazil nuts).

Wheat*

White Or Whole Wheat?

The human equivalent of "fake" food is white flour. 98% of spaghetti, bread, pastries, and pancakes are made with white flour. Such products can be caramel colored to make you think you are eating 100% whole wheat products. Wheat and sprouted wheat may taste similar, but they are two completely dissimilar foods. This is why so many people are recommending eating only sprouted breads. In the milling (or grinding) process there is a significant amount of heat generated that has a harmful effect on the grain. Nearly all milling oxidizes the kernel, losing critical vitamins, including Vitamin E, within 24 hours. Most of the bran and germ is removed in the milling process. By removing these ingredients it allows most flours, including whole wheat, to have a longer shelf life. The flour (void of many nutrients) will last for several months on the store shelf without going rancid.

Zinc Deficiency

White flour products are missing 62% of the zinc found in whole wheat. Is it any wonder that half of Americans are zinc deficient? Zinc is a part of every living cell and is essential for the activity of over 200 biological enzymes. It is critical for normal hormonal activity and a healthy immune system.

Magnesium Deficiency

Three out of four Americans don't have enough magnesium in their diet. White flour is missing 72% compared to whole wheat. Magnesium is a must in over 300 enzyme activities, especially the production of ATP (which helps supply energy to every part of your body). It is a must for a healthy heart!

Magnesium dilates arteries and bronchial passages. When added to calcium intake it is 16 times more effective at promoting bone density than calcium alone!

Benefits Of Sprouted Wheat

A superior way to get the most available nutrients from grain is either to stone grind it yourself and use it within 24 hours, or, if you want to be way ahead health-wise and have enhanced nutrients, more vitamins and enzymes, and change the bread from an acid to an alkaline base, sprout it. The sprouting process causes a polysaccharide change in the kernel, rendering it to be an allergically friendly food. As the wheat sprouts the starch in the grain starts turning to maltose to feed the shoot.

Malted (Sprouted) Wheat Vs. Non-Malted Wheat

According to research undertaken at the University of Minnesota, sprouting increases the total nutrient density.

Riboflavin (vitamin B2) increase of 315%.
Vitamin C increase of 300%.
Folic Acid increase of 278%.
Biotin increase of 111%.
Niacin (Vitamin B3) increase of 66%.
Pantothenic Acid (Vitamin B5) increase of 65%.
Thiamine (Vitamin B1) increase of 28%.

Not only did sprouting increase the available vitamins for absorption, but also significantly increases various enzymes, including amylase, protease and lipase. All grains undergo this type of quantitative and qualitative transformation.

Stop The Bread Craving

Folks that have been eating mostly raw, living food have found that their cravings for bread have diminished tremendously. Most Americans eat some type of bread at every meal and snack. Like muffins/toast for breakfast, sandwiches for lunch, and rolls or biscuits with dinner. Bread is an American staple. But raw food followers tell me they never thought they would be saying this, but, "They don't miss bread." That's right, they don't miss their bread and they get all their nutrients, too.

The Trouble With Gluten

"Gluten, the sticky, difficult to digest wheat protein, breaks down during germination. Other changes are the destruction of phytic and oxalic acids. (Oxalic acid binds to calcium causing the most common form of kidney stones-calcium oxalate stones). These acids bind up minerals like phosphorus, calcium and zinc," says Steve Meyerowitz in an article entitled, "Sprout Route," in Alive Magazine. So, the bulk of the gluten in breads is contained in the wheat germ and once sprouted, it breaks down, making breads more digestible.

So How Do You Sprout Wheat?

Soak your seeds and grains for about 8 hours. Soaking them overnight is convenient. Put 3-4 tablespoons of seeds in your sprouting/soaking container and cover generously with purified water. At the end of 8 hours, or when you get up in the morning, thoroughly drain the seeds/grain. Rise the seeds/grain for about 30 seconds under rushing tap water. This is a very important step. Rinsing your seeds with purified water doesn't give enough volume and pressure to rinse the seeds thoroughly. After rinsing your seeds, make sure you drain or shake off any excess water. If your seeds are in excess water they will rot. When your seeds have been soaked, rinsed and drained once, they will begin sprouting. Continue rinsing and draining three times daily (once in the morning, once in the afternoon and once in the evening) for about 3 days or till the seeds have sprouted (a tail).

Sprouted Wheat Bread Recipe

This bread recipe is so simple I even did it. Why is it so simple? It's bread made from one ingredient!

1 cup wheat (seeds) berries
Sprouting container
Food processor with S blade
Small Pyrex type bowl (heat resistant)
Crock-pot with low setting

Follow the sprouting directions above. Soak your wheat berries eight hours or overnight. Then rinse and drain the berries three times a day for the next 32 hours or until the wheat berries have sprouted ¼ inch tails. Important: Make sure the berries are well drained before processing into dough. In other words, don't rinse after they are finished sprouting! Place the sprouted wheat berries into your food processor with the S blade in place and pulse until the berries resemble bread dough and form a ball around the food processor blade. No added liquid is required. Remove the ball of dough from the food processor. Shape the dough into 1 small ball. You may want to sprinkle with freshly ground corn meal. Place the shaped dough into a small Pyrex type bowl that will easily fit into your crock pot. Place the cover on your crock-pot and turn to its lowest setting. Cook the bread for approximately 8 hours or until the bread is a rich, dark brown. The top of the bread may crack and it will have a tough, thick crust on the outside and a moist, brown bread on the inside. This recipe will serve about 4. It will stay fresh in your refrigerator for about 1 week.

*Those with true celiac disease (allergy to wheat) should avoid any wheat products.

References:

The Rice Stuff, www.menshealth.com. May 2001:32

Kayahara, H., American Chemical Society, 2001.

Paulen, G.B., "The Divine Philosophy And Science Of Health And Healing," Teach Services, Brushton, NY, 1995:129-130.

Crisafi, D.J., "Sprouting Grains," Alive Magazine, Aug. 1995. Silver Hills Bakery, www.silverhillsbakery.com, 2008. www.exhealthydiet.com/sprouted-grain-bread.html 2008. www.exhealthydiet.com/sprouts.html 2008.

CHARCOAL

- Nature's Purifier

*Fomentations of pulverized charcoal, in a porous bag, placed on one's back and stomach has been shown, to bring relief of spasms and pain in as little as 30 min.**

Charcoal Uses In And Out Of The Human Body

2000 BCE**, ancient Egyptian doctors used charcoal poultices for fever, snake bites, insects stings, inflammation of the bowels, to filter water, to eliminate odors and relieves gas pains. Charcoal adsorbs more poisons than any other substance known to man. It can adsorb thousands of times its own weight in gases, heavy metals and poisons. It has been shown to adsorb arsenic, DDT, drugs (like codeine, Tylenol, penicillin, aspirin, phenobarbital etc), inorganic substances (chlorine, lead, mercury, fluoride, etc), poison ivy, snake bites, mushroom poisoning, brown recluse spider bites, black widow bites, to name a few.

The Ultimate Antidote

Scientific experiments attest to the effectiveness of charcoal as an antidote. In one experiment, 100 times the lethal dose of cobra venom was mixed with charcoal and injected into lab animals. The animals were not harmed. 1831, a French pharmacist, swallowed charcoal at the same time that he took strychnine to show that charcoal was an effective remedy for all poisons. He died — of old age. Using charcoal does not relieve you of your responsibility to seek medical attention if poisoned! If poisoned, induce vomiting first, then give the charcoal. Never give charcoal to an unconscious person. Poison Hot Line 1 800 222-1222.

Activated Charcoal

Today specially processed or Activated charcoal is used to treat poisoning and overdoses in the Emergency Room, adsorbing thousands of times its own weight in gases, heavy metals and poisons, rendering them ineffective and harmless. Unlike regular charcoal, Activated charcoal has an extremely large surface area. One teaspoonful has the surface area of more than 10,000 square feet (1000 square meters per gram). Thus, activated charcoal can readily adsorb or bind toxins from within (stomach and intestines) or on the skin (bites, stings, pimples, infections). In an acute poisoning it is not unusual to give 3 cups (200 grams) of activated charcoal, repeated every four hours or till one's stool turns black.

Where Does Charcoal Come From?

Activated charcoal can come from incompletely burned hard wood, coconut shells, bamboo, olive pits or coal (Lignite or Anthracite). It is a very fine or granular, black, odorless, tasteless powder. Medical use Activated Charcoal USP (U.S. Pharmacopoeia) is wood charcoal carbon that is free from inorganic material, contains less than 4% ash residue and has no carcinogenic properties.

Charcoal to Avoid – Charcoal from burned toast or other burned foods contains carcinogenic substances-avoid this type of charcoal. Never ingest charcoal briquettes because they contain petroleum products.

How I Make It

One can start with crushed charcoal tablets or powdered activated charcoal. Take equal parts charcoal and ground flaxseed or corn starch with just enough hot water to make a paste. Place it between two layers of wax paper and roll it out thin with rolling pin. We make it ahead of time as a family project. Then place in the freezer to take out and break off pieces to use as needed. The flaxseed/corn starch is optional but makes it easier to handle. Sometimes we make it fresh as a paste and place it between two layers of porous cloth and secure it to the needed body part for up to 10 hours or all night. Keep your container of charcoal closed tightly because it will collect all the room impurities before you get to use it.

Who Needs It?

I have found a warning label on a few brands of charcoal, saying not to be given to infants, children, pregnant women or nursing women. If this is pure activated charcoal USP, there is no restriction on age or gender for its use.

Why Use It?

Any area on your body that is red, painful, swollen and hot responds to charcoal. Place a moist warm poultice compress on the site. Charcoal actually draws bacteria, toxins and poisons through the skin and into the poultice. Here's an example: For a red infection around a wound: make a charcoal poultice and place it over the inflamed site, cover with plastic wrap to prevent the charcoal from getting on your clothes. Remember this could stain/tattoo your skin black temporarily. The only reason I mention this is one of my girls (which one will remain nameless) about 10 years ago placed some on her face to clear up her skin. She was horrified when we insisted that she go to church that week. Isn't makeup wonderful!

Diabetic Ulcer/Bedsores:

I've seen non-healing diabetic ulcers of the feet (not responding to antibiotics and recommended for amputation) respond to charcoal poultices. The feet were placed in plastic bags filled with a mixture of charcoal and water and changed four times a day, until better. This also works well for stubborn decubitus bedsores that won't heal.

Too Much Gas/Bad Breath

Charcoal reduces the amount of gas produced (upper and lower) after eating beans and other gas forming foods. It also adsorbs the bacteria which forms the gas. Activated charcoal helps resolve bad breath by adsorbing bacteria and volatile breath odors.

Diarrhea

Charcoal relieves nervous diarrhea, traveler's diarrhea, spastic colon, indigestion, and helps heal peptic ulcers. You may use charcoal tablets or take one to two tablespoons of powdered charcoal mixed with olive oil, swirl in a glass of water and drink. Take three times a day or if one has severe diarrhea, every hour until it is resolved. Take charcoal between meals because food decreases its effectiveness. Remember to re-hydrate and replace your trace minerals/electrolytes after using charcoal, (like a tomato juice product or sports drink). I don't recommend taking charcoal daily because it adsorbs all your vitamins, prescription meds, minerals and nutrients.

Pets

Yes, the family pet can be benefitted too by charcoal, given either internally or externally, for the itch, infected skin, the runs, or poisoning.

* White, E.G., Selected Messages, Vol.2, 294-5
** BCE=Before Common Era

References:
"Amazing Charcoal," http://www.sdadefend.com/MINDEX-C.htm.
Paulien, G.B., *"Charcoal,"* The Divine Philosophy And Science Of Health And Healing, TEACH Services. 1995.
Poison Hot Line Web Page http://www.aapcc.org/DNN/ 1 800 222-1222
"Amazing Charcoal" Lancet , 09-13-80
Baldwin, M., Wildwood Sanitarium and Hospital, Wildwood, GA.
http://www.tpministries.org/charcoal.htm
Other Health Nuggets: ParkRidgeCardiology.com

THE CHOLESTEROL MYTH

- Inflammation Causes Heart Disease, Not Cholesterol

"A new heart also will I give you, and a new spirit will I put within you: and I will take away the stony heart out of your flesh, and I will give you an heart of flesh." Ezekiel 36:26

Heart Attacks

Someone has a heart attack every 30 seconds in the U.S. Each year over a million people in the U.S. have a heart attack. About half of them die. Many people have permanent heart damage or die because they don't get help immediately. It's important to know the symptoms of a heart attack and call 911 if someone is having them. Those symptoms include: chest discomfort/pressure, squeezing, or pain; shortness of breath; discomfort in the upper body/ arms, jaw, shoulder, neck or back; nausea, vomiting, dizziness, lightheadedness or sweating. These symptoms can sometimes be different in women. What exactly is a heart attack? Most heart attacks happen when a clot/scab in the coronary artery blocks the supply of blood and oxygen to the heart. Often this leads to an irregular heartbeat (called an arrhythmia), that causes a severe decrease in the pumping function of the heart. A complete blockage that is not treated within a few hours causes the affected heart muscle to die.

Is All Cholesterol Bad?

Cholesterol is an essential component of cell membranes (walls). It also is required for the synthesis of estrogen, testosterone, adrenaline, cortisone, vitamin D and other hormones; as well as being one component in your bile acids that helps digest your fats. Even "bad" low density lipoprotein-LDL cholesterol is necessary for optimal health. Babies need cholesterol rich foods for development of their brains and nervous systems. We all have a genetically determined amount of cholesterol we produce. The problem is we eat extra cholesterol in cholesterol rich foods, which adds to our risk of disease and to our cholesterol number.

Free Radicals

Free radicals are chemical by-products of many reactions within the body called "oxidation. They are called "free" in the sense that they damage cells, tissue and processes in the body without adequate control. People eat too much food that is oxidized or easily oxidized and it ends up in the wrong place, like the arteries of your heart. Researchers now understand how the arteries become plugged with lipid (fatty) material. Cooked cholesterol (only found in animal products) foods cause oxidation (rusting) of the blood vessel lining. An example is when butter is left out of the refrigerator for as little as 20 minutes, it oxidizes. Then you wonder how you got heart disease. High fat, low fiber, high sugar diets (fast food or processed foods) promote oxidation. Free radical damage may be caused by cell toxins like tobacco and alcohol and a faulty response to stress; which adds even more to the risk of oxidation.

Trans Fats

Trans fats (anything hydrogenated, including hydrogenated soy) promotes the worst oxidation. New government labeling allows a product to place on its label "no trans fats" if it contains less than ½ gram of trans fats per serving. Thus, if there is 10 servings in a package, there could be 5 grams of hidden trans fat in that product. Look on the ingredients label to see if it says the word 'hydrogenated.' If it does, avoid it.

Your Cholesterol Particle Size

So you can make a difference by your diet in the type of cholesterol particles you have (fluffy beach balls-good or dense sand-bad). In some of my patients their cholesterol numbers (total cholesterol, HDL, LDL, VLDL, triglycerides) do not change significantly with diet and exercise and this causes them to be discouraged. Have your doctor check the cholesterol particle size and number after your aggressive diet change. You will see a big difference. The larger the particle (HDL and LDL), the less likely it will abrasion and get lodged between cells, starting the inflammation process in your arteries. Current studies reflex a closer correlation for risk of coronary artery disease with the Non HDL Chol number than the LDL number. Non HDL Chol is your total cholesterol number minus your HDL number.

Saturated Fat

Contrary to popular belief, saturated fats do not cause heart disease. Saturated fat can be made by your body into cholesterol, so moderation in all things applies here. We need saturated fats, which are necessary for calcium to be incorporated into our bones. Omega-3 fats are retained better in tissues in the presence of saturated fats. Saturated fats promote healthy immune systems because of their anti-microbial properties that prevent the buildup of harmful micro-organisms in the digestive tract. Some of the best sources of saturated fat are nuts. Omega-3 fats are found in walnuts, pecans and brazil nuts.

Diet Changes For Better Cholesterol Numbers

Eat more fresh fruits (especially blueberries) and veggies (red veggies are high in Vitamin C). Eat more nuts, like walnuts (omega-3) and almonds (magnesium). Eat more seeds (for zinc and complete natural Vitamin E), like sunflower seeds and pumpkin seeds. Cook with extra virgin olive oil (made from the first pressing of ripe olives) containing oleic acid, a heart friendly cooking oil. Avoid cholesterol containing foods (meat, eggs, cheese and milk) which raise your cholesterol.

The Side Effects Of Statin Drugs

Cholesterol drugs, called statins, lower the bad LDL cholesterol and thus reduce heart attacks by as much as 50% and stroke by as much as 25%. They have, as does any drug, side-effects which include: muscle damage (rare), permanent liver damage (rarer), headaches, upset stomach muscle aches and rashes. Don't take statins with grapefruit or its juice, because it increases the drug concentration and the risk of side-effects (even if you take a statin 24 hours after eating grapefruit). The statins work by limiting (amount depends on the specific drug) the product of cholesterol in the liver. Statins also reduce the production of CoEnzQ10, which may cause many of its side-effects. Lack of CoEnzQ10 can increase your toxic level of homocyteine. I recommend 100 mg ofCoEnzQ10 a day while taking any statins. Another reason, I believe, some people can't take statin drugs is that their body's acid base balance is too acidic. Eating a more alkaline diet (the healthiest) suddenly allows these people to be able to take a statin drugs without side effects.

The Real Reason Statin May Benefit You

But the reason statins reduce the incidence of heart disease may not be from their cholesterol effects at all, but is probably from their powerful anti-inflammatory and anti-oxidant effects that prevent cell and tissue damage. This is the reason they are being recommended to patients with diabetes and rheumatoid arthritis with normal cholesterol levels. You've heard the bad things about statins, what about the good things statin do?

Alzheimer's Disease

Large observational studies have shown statins to lower the risk of Alzheimer's disease by 30-70% and delays its onset. True Alzheimer's is from a build up of amyloid proteins in the brain causing a glue-liken on dissolvable plaque. The immune system detects these plaques and releases inflammatory molecules to destroy it. Continued attack on the cells causes damage to the surrounding brain cells without breaking down the plaque. Statins don't help in Alzheimer's by lowering the cholesterol number, but by reducing the inflammation that causes the damage to the brain.

Parkinsonism

Analysis of data of 1,684,810 patients showed a 49% reduction in the incidence of Parkinsonism when the patents took Zocor (simvastatin), but not Lipitor (avorvastatin) or Mevacor/Red Rice Yeast (lovastatin).

Cancer

Several studies have shown statins reduce colon cancer by 50%, prostate cancer by 56%, melanomas and breast cancer by 30%. Statins block the activation of an enzyme complex (proteasome) that break down proteins and thus block the growth of cancer cells. Statins may also block cell signals that can trigger continuous cancer cell division.

Glaucoma

Statins help improve the nutrition in the eye by improved circulation and this then promotes better drainage, which lowers the pressure in the eye. Men that had been on statins for over two years had 40% less glaucoma and had a reduced risk of developing age related macular degeneration (which is the number one cause of blindness in people overage 65 in the U.S.).

Rheumatoid Arthritis

Statins reduce the rheumatoid arthritis flares, C-reactive protein and swollen joints after six months of treatment. Women with rheumatoid arthritis for at least 10 years increased their risk of a heart attack threefold. So even if your cholesterol numbers are OK, you may want to consider a statin.

Diabetes

The American Diabetes Association strongly suggests taking a statin as part of a complete treatment plan. Their guidelines recommend that diabetics over the age of 40 with a total cholesterol greater than 135 take a statin for the anti-inflammatory/cholesterol effect, because diabetics have a higher risk of silent heart attack and stroke.

Non-Statin Prescription Cholesterol Reduction

Other ways to lower your cholesterol number besides statins, diet and exercise include prescription: cholestyramine (Questran, Cholestid), niacin (Niaspan), fibrates (Lofibrate, Tricor, Antara, Lopid), omega-3 (Lovaza, formerly known as Omacor), Welchol and Zetia.

Natural Ways To Lower Your Cholesterol

Many people can reduce their cholesterol numbers by cutting out animal products (meat, eggs, milk and cheese), exercising, avoiding products made with coconut and palm oils, and eating more fiber (oat bran, oatmeal and raw foods, etc). Few people can lower their "bad" cholesterol number to the recommended level (70 or below), for those at high risk, without a statin drug (Lipitor, Caduet, Vytorin, Crestor, Zocor, Pravastatin, Lescol, Levostatin, Mevacor, etc.). Natural herb remedies for cholesterol do lower the cholesterol number some, but do they change the particle size of the cholesterol components? The literature is not clear on this relatively new issue.

Best Cholesterol Lowering Herbs

Here are some suggestions for reducing your LDL cholesterol via supplements. There are over fifty on the internet. Start with one supplement at a time, adding others one by one, until your desired LDL is met. Unfortunately, long-term use of any herb can be as toxic as prescription meds and just as costly. See your health care professional before starting any herbal program!!!

Artichoke (Cynara scolymus), taken as a tincture with water three times a day, lowers LDL "bad" cholesterol by almost 23%.

Garlic (Allium sativum), two to four raw cloves daily, chopped up and added at the end of cooking or to salads, lowers LDL by 11.4% and increases particle size.

Guggul (Commiphora mukul), one 25mg cap three times a day until cholesterol is normal. Guggul lowers LDL by 12.5%. Not for long term use. All three herbs can be taken together. Take them for at least two weeks to see results.

Tocotrienols, alpha, beta, delta, gamma, are forms of vitamin E. Take

200mg at dinner. Any other vitamin E supplement should be taken in the morning, so that it doesn't interfere with the tocotrienols. Good sources of vitamin E include all seeds (pumpkin and sunflower) and almonds.

Policosanol/guggulipid. It is a sugarcane extract/herb combination. Take 500 mg with breakfast and dinner.

Policosanol and vitamin E have a blood thinning effect. Don't use them if you regularly use aspirin, plavix, other non-steroidal anti-inflammatories (NSAIDs), (like Aleve, Motrin, etc) or warfarin (coumadin).

Inositol hexaniacinate, a timed release niacin that, unlike other niacin supplements, does not cause flushing and is not toxic to the liver. Take 600 mg with each meal (3x/day).

Red Rice Yeast is nature's "statin" and is levostatin (identical to Mevacor). Take two 600 mg tabs twice a day. You must watch for muscle aching and liver abnormalities just like a prescription statin. The side effects are the same as prescription statins.

References:

"Heart Attack," National Heart, Lung, and Blood Institute

BottomLine, *"Your Diet,"* and *"These Cholesterol Drugs,"* August 1,2004:16 and December 1, 2004:9-11.

Sica, R., *"Natural Ways To Lower Your Cholesterol,"* Bottom Line, October 15, 2004; 2.

Neustaadter, R, *"The Cholesterol Myth,"* Letsliveonline.com, Feb 2005:22.

"Your Guide To Great Living," Letsliveonline.com, Feb 2005:38-40. http:// www. Prevention.com

Fotuhi, M., *"The Memory Cure: How To Protect Your Brain Against Memory Loss And Alzheimer's Disease,"* McGraw Hill, 2002.

Marks, S., *"Prostate And Cancer,"* Perseus, 2002.

Abel, R. Jr, *"The Eye Care Revolution,"* Kensington, 1999.

New England Journal Of Medicine, *"Statins And Cancer,"* May 26,2005:online edition.

Wolozin, B, *"Superior Results With Longterm Zocor,"* BioMed Central (BMC) Medicine. Reported in BottomLine 10/1/07:7.

DEPRESSION IS NOT A DRUG DEFICIENCY

- What Can You Do To Prevent Depression?
- The Black Hole Of Depression
- 27 Million In The US Use Antidepressants!

A Look Into How We Think

The majority of my patients have a mood disorder, depression being the most common. More than 10% of the population is treated for depression. Depression is predictably a complex problem. There is no "standard" case of depression. It can stem from numerous forms of stress, inherited and cultivated pathways in our brains and from bad habits. Our heavenly Father has made our bodies to have an innate capability to cope, repair and function without self-destructing. Emotional, physical or chemical triggers can disrupt our brain chemistry. There are over 5000 known chemicals in the human brain that function to keep us stable and alive. Any one of them that is not delivered to its receptor properly can cause you to be unbalanced, and the devil knows this.

SSRIs

Over the last 20 years, a family of drugs called Selective Serotonin Reuptake Inhibitors (SSRIs)* have become the most popularly prescribed medicine in the world. SSRIs are used for mild to moderate depression (not bipolar depression or major depression). SSRIs increase serotonin levels in the brain and are safer than the tricyclic antidepressants discovered in the 1950's. Every medication comes with a very long list of side effects. Any medication can cause any side effect in any given patient at any time. Antidepressants have been shown to be only moderately effective, so what else can I do?

Serotonin

Serotonin is a chemical neurotransmitter (the happy brain chemical) that helps relay electrical signals from one neuron to another between the cell ends (synapses). Only 10% of serotonin is manufactured in the brain where it has various functions, including control of appetite, sleep, mood and anger. 90% of our serotonin supply is found in the digestive tract, where it is used to regulate intestinal movements and in blood platelets. In fact, every important chemical in our brain has an identical chemical structure counter part in our human gut.

Tryptophan

Serotonin is made via a unique biochemical conversion process using tryptophan, a protein building block, which forms 5-hydoxytryptamine

(5-HT), otherwise known as serotonin. Tryptophan is one of 20 essential amino acids in the human diet. Essential amino acids are not manufacture by mammals, who must eat enough to supply their needs. Tryptophan is encoded in the standard genetic DNA code as the codon UGG. Tryptophan is a routine constituent of most protein-based foods. Plant based sources are alkaline (not acidic) and are the best source of tryptophan. Tryptophan is found in: chocolate, oats, durians, mangoes, dried dates, milk, yogurt, cottage cheese, eggs, sesame, chickpeas, sunflower seeds, pumpkin seeds, spirulina, walnuts, almonds, tofu, gluten flour and peanuts. Complex carbohydrates (rice, potato, pasta) may increase serotonin levels some, explaining feel good carbohydrate comfort foods, but the protein content of these foods might actually inhibit serotonin production over time. Although tryptophan is found in red meat, fish and poultry, it competes with other essential amino acids** flowing to the brain tissue. Therefore, the human body must get enough tryptophan from other sources to make enough serotonin to prevent one getting depressed (serotonin depleted).

Sugar And Serotonin

Harmful dietary habits that increase serotonin levels temporarily are, believe it or not, candy and sweets, which are simple carbohydrates. Sugar has the greatest impact on serotonin levels, but only increases serotonin for one to two hours. This may explain the Candy/Chocolate craving so many of my patients have. This has a yo-yo effect on their mood by creating wildly fluctuating serotonin levels in their gut and brain. No wonder they come to me depressed!!!

Herbals For Mood St John's Wort

St. John's Wort-Hypericum Perforatum is a shrub perennial used for mild and moderate depression (not bipolar depression or major depression and not to be combined with other SSRIs). Its mechanism of action is illusive, but it is believed to lie in selective inhibition of serotonin, dopamine and norepinephrine re-uptake in the central nervous system. Its active compounds are hypericin and hyperforin. Multiple studies have shown an over 50% improvement in symptoms. St John's Wort can cause photo sensitivity and cataracts. Consult with your Care Giver to be sure there are no contraindications with other prescriptions you might be taking.

SAMe

"Sammy", SAMe, S-adenosyl-methionine is a natural occurring brain chemical that provides a boost to both mood and outlook. It is formed from the essential amino acid methionine and adenosine triphosphate

(ATP). Approved in the US in 1999, it is thought to increase the neurotransmitters serotonin, dopamine and norepinephrine.

5-Hydroxytryptophan (5-HTP)

The seeds of an African plant--Griffonia simplicifolia, are the precursor of serotonin. It is metabolized in the small bowel, increasing levels of serotonin in the brain by 5-HTP being decarboxylated to serotonin (5-hydroxytryptamine or 5-HT) by the enzyme aromatic-L-amino-acid decarboxylase with the help of Vitamin B6. This over the counter supplement "Tryptophan" (5-HTP) was banned from sale in the US in 1991 for 38 deaths and 1500 having a disabling autoimmune illness called eosinophilia-myalgia syndrome (EMS). It was traced to a contaminant (Peak-X) in L-tryptophan supplied by the Japanese manufacturer, Showa Denko. Since 2002, L-tryptophan (5-HTP) has been sold in the U.S. in its original form.

Other Mood Improving Herbs

Chamomile has been used for depressed mood and loss of appetite. Feverfew can be helpful for migraines and lifting the spirit. Ginkgo Biloba can increase blood flow to the brain, if lack of blood flow is the cause, thus improving your mood. Lavender and its aroma can improve the mood, nervousness and insomnia. Lemon Balm can improve nervousness, insomnia and gastric complaints. Valerian can help nervousness, insomnia, stress and anxiety.

Food For Mood
Omega-3

Omega 3 benefits eye problems and inflammatory diseases because it inhibits prostaglandin E2 (PE2). PE2 contributes to blood vessel inflammation and plaque on arteries. Other anti-inflammatory processes which may be helped include: arthritis, cancer, Crohn's disease, diabetes, Alzheimer's disease, peripheral neuropathy, psoriasis, cardiac dysrrhythmias (atrial and ventricular), PMS, mood disorders and depression to name a few.

Flaxseed, a source of Omega-3 fatty acids (alpha linolenic acid-ALA) and lignan, has been shown to inhibit melanoma, breast cancer and prostate cancer growth. Two tablespoons of freshly ground flaxseed a day decreased free testosterone and cholesterol levels, by day 21-43. Low-grade prostate disease had a decreased cell proliferation in the flaxseed groups, but a recent study of 47,000 men showed that flaxseed oil may worsen advanced prostate cancer. The reason was high levels of ALA did not convert to the beneficial EPA/DHA Omega-3. EPA (eicosapentaenoic acid) and DHA (docosahexaenoic acid) are polyunsaturated fatty acids that are part of the omega-3 family and are found in cold water fish. The enzyme delta six desaturase converts ALA (vegetarian sources) to EPA/DHA, but delta six desaturase is severely inhibited by elevated insulin levels. Thus, anyone with diabetes type 2 that is over weight, having high cholesterol or high blood pressure can have elevated insulin levels and should not take vegetarian sources for their omega 3, but use fish oil (the only direct source of EPA/DHA)! Omega 3 (alpha linolenic acid-ALA) is found in:

Flaxseed 1 Tbs 7520 mg., English walnuts 1/4 cup 2043 mg., Canola oil 1 Tbsp 1267 mg., Black walnuts 1/4 cup 1031 mg., Wheat germ oil 1 Tbs 938 mg., Soybean oil 1 Tbs 927 mg., Green soybeans 1 cup 637 mg., Spinach (canned) 1 cup 353 mg., Avocados ½ cup 132 mg., Almonds 1/4 cup 127 mg., Safflower oil 1 Tbs 55 mg., Turnips 1 cup 50 mg., Banana (medium) 39 mg., Sweet potatoes 1 cup 36 mg., Apple (medium) 25 mg., Potato (medium) 17 mg., Cucumber ½ cup 16 mg., Whole Wheat bread 14 mg., Omega 6 essential amino acid (gamma linolenic acid-GLA is the isomer of ALA)., Borage Oil, Evening Primrose Oil, Black currant seed oil, Hemp seeds, Spirulina, All GLA should be cold pressed

Homocysteine

Your homocysteine level helps predict how fast you will age, your B vitamin-nutritional status, your immune-system function, and the state of your brain. It also helps show how well your body's chemistry can roll with life's stresses. Your body forms homocysteine when you eat any animal or vegetable protein, because it contains the amino acid methionine. But too much homocysteine (like a high protein diet or life long protein only diet-including a typical diet of only meat and potatoes) literally shreds your arteries from the inside out, allowing fat and cholesterol to stick to the walls of your blood vessels. Our blood level of homocysteine is more accurate than your cholesterol number in predicting the risk of a heart attack, stroke or Alzheimer's disease.

Thirty years of research has shown that excess homocysteine disables a mechanism in your arterial cells called contact inhibition. Contact inhibition regulates the growth of the smooth muscle cells just below the endothelium (inner wall) of your arteries. This causes smooth muscle cells to multiply out of control, creating a bulge that pushes other layers of the vessel wall apart and causes protrusions into the artery. Your body requires a steady supply of a particular "helper nutrient," to process, convert and excrete excess homocysteine–B Vitamins. These

B vitamins help convert homocysteine into harmless cystathione and methionine. Folic acid is the most important B vitamin in controlling your homocysteine levels. There are over 800 studies demonstrating folic acids' benefit in fighting homocysteine. All nine of the "B" vitamins (Thiamine B1, riboflavin B2, niacin B3, pyridoxine B6, biotin, inositol, p-aminobenzoic acid PABA, cyanocobalamin B12, and folic acid) are found in citrus fruits, spinach, asparagus, broccoli, Brussel sprouts and fresh leafy green veggies (more below). Blueberries are one of the highest sources of folic acid in a fruit/berry. You need at least nine servings a day if your homocysteine levels are high. Also remember: high levels of folic acid can mask a B12 deficiency and avoid "B" supplements if you have just had a bare metal coronary stent placed. B vitamins are OK with drug eluding stents. The bare metal stent has been shown to close down faster when people were taking B6, B12 and folic acid vitamins, but not when eating foods high in "B" vitamins.

Folic Acid Deficiency

Folic acid deficiency can be a direct cause of depression. It is more commonly seen in meat eaters.

Sources of Folic Acid:

Chickpeas 1 cup - 1114 mcg., Black-eyed Cowpeas 1 cup - 1057 mcg., Lentils 1 cup - 831 mcg., Red Kidney Beans 1 cup - 725 mcg., Okra pods 1 cup - 269 mcg., Navy Beans 1 cup - 255 mcg., Spinach 1 cup - 109 mcg., Mustard greens 1 cup - 105 mcg., Spanish Peanuts 1/4 cup - 88 mcg., Fresh Orange Juice 1 cup - 75 mcg.

B12 Deficiency

B12 deficiency is much more common than previously thought. Since B12 accelerates the synaptic function of your nerves, it can directly cause fatigue and depression.

Sources of B12 include:

Dry cereal (Total) 3 oz - 6 mcg., Fortified breads 1 slice - 1 mcg., Egg 1 large - 1 mcg., Soy milk 8 oz -1 mcg., Skim milk 8 oz . -38 mcg., Nutritional (Brewer's) yeast 1 tsp - 1.2 mcg., Seaweed products 1/4 cup .002 mcg., Spinach organic 1 cup - .02 mcg.
Soybean organic 1 cup - .01 mcg.
Skin of potatoes .01 – mcg.
Fruits and vegetables - NONE

Heavy Metal Toxicity

Lead, mercury, arsenic, bismuth, organotins, trimethyltin chloride, solvents (like carbondisulfide, toluene, perchloroethyleneand trichloroethylene) can cause depression, fibromyalgia and mooddisorders. The most common sources of lead includes: drinking water, dust, calcium supplements (usually from China), manufacturing environments and lead based paint. Mercury sources include: imported herbs and vitamins, beauty supplies, certain vaccines, and fish (including fish oil capsules). The most common source for arsenic poisoning is chicken. Arsenic is used prior to processing to kill the bird's parasites. The chronic use of Pepto-Bismol can cause gray matter changes of your brain, thus mood disorders. Organotins (and organophosphates) are from insect and rodent killers and disinfectants. Industrial workers can show signs of a mood disorder due to various solvent exposures. Heavy metal testing at your Care Provider is available.

Low Thyroid (Hypothyroid)

40% of the US population have an underactive thyroid which can cause depression, fatigue, dry skin, hair loss and brain fog. Fluoride (water supplies, tooth care products), a high intake of soy (not tofu or tempeh) and bromide (sodas, breads etc) have been shown to interfere with iodine metabolism and thus inhibit thyroid function. A gluten free diet can help those with thyroid antibodies (Hashimoto's Thyroiditis, Graves' Disease). I recommend a blood test including: TSH, Free T3, Free T4 and thyroid antibodies. Using a prescription thyroid to bring your blood levels up to high normal can improve your mood.

Other Causes Of Depression

Lack of exercise, any chronic health problem, lack of sleep, legal (nicotine and alcohol) and illegal drug use, absence of social support, caffeine (and theobromine = chocolate, tea), in between meal snacking, movies, TV, video games, internet, high sugar intake, lack of trace minerals–like magnesium, etc. Self help for depression, once you are in the black hole is rarely helpful. Turning to your friends, care provider and family may be your only solution.

Changes You Can Make

1. Eat a low-fat vegetarian diet, rich in fresh fruits and vegetables.

2. Exercising in the sunlight, markedly improved depression in 75% of the cases.

3. Music therapy (it worked for King Saul). Rock music has been shown to contribute to depression.

4. Regular restful sleep. Correcting a sleeping disorder can improve chronic pain and your mood.

5. Inner spiritual experience. Daily devotions lift the mood. Nothing tends to promote health of body and soul more than a spirit of gratitude and praise. "Think Happy."

6. Avoid anger; it can cause depression.

7. Social support (own a pet). As Christians we can play a part in supporting those around us.

8. Hydrotherapy, massage, etc.

9. Three Steps: Analysis of your life, a desire to change, the courage to embark on a new plan for your life.

10. Nutrition and lifestyle choices offer a reasonable expectation of a lasting solution to mood disorders.

Help For Depression

Isaiah 58:10,11- Service to others gives peace.
Proverbs 17:22 - Keep a smile on your heart.
Matthew 6:34; Philippians 4:6 - Don't worry.
1 Thessalonians 5: 16-18; Phil 4:4-7 - Rejoice, pray with thanks.
Isaiah 26:3; Psalm 40:1-4 - For peace, focus on Christ.

*Citalopram (Celexa), Escitalopram (Lexapro), Fluoxetine (Prozac), Paroxetine (Paxil, Paxil CR, Pexeva), Sertraline (Zoloft), Fluvoxamine (Luvox)
**Tyrosine, Valine, Isoleucine, Leucine, Phenylalanine, and other large neutral amino acids

References:

Barbara, P., *"Antidepressant Use Doubles In US, Study Says,"* Reuters, Aug 3, 2009.

Nedley, N, *"Depression, The Way Out,"* 2001, Nedley Publishing,Ardmore, OK.

Williams, D., *"Depression Is Not A Drug Deficiency,"* Alternatives, April 2008; 73-80.

Lucca, A., *"Plasma tryptophan levels and plasma tryptophan/neutralamino acid ratio in patients with mood disorder, patients with obsessivecompulsive disorder, and normal subjects,"* Psychiatry 1995 Jul;9(4):615-626.

The Failure Of Flaxseed To Reduce Prostate Cancer. Am J Clin Nutr, July 2004;80(1):204-216.

15,000 Physicians And Their Homocysteine Levels, Harvard Study, JAMA, 1992; Vol.268, 877-881.

"Folic Acid And Stents Don't Mix," Cardiology News, Aug 2003:16.

Birdsall TC, "5-Hydroxytryptophan: a clinically-effective serotonin precursor" Alternative Medicine Review: Journal of Clinical Therapeutic August 1998;3 (4): 271-80.

Wilson, J., *"Hypothyroidism: Lacking In Metabolic Fire,"* Health Matters, Vol.1, Iss.6, HYPERLINK "http://www.parkridgecardiology.com/, http:/www. gsmcweb.com/www. gsmcweb.com.

FLUORIDE

- A deficient diet, not a fluoride deficiency, is the cause of most dental decay.

After rigorous inquiry and with sound scientific, legalistic, and ethical reasons, I find fluoride to be ...., **Now you decide!**

Fluoride's Benefits

Fluoride is known as the champion cavity fighter. Fluoride products help strengthen children's teeth at ages 9 to 12, but the American Dental Association in 2007 issued a warning that fluoridated water should not be used in infant formulas or foods. 66% of US cities and towns have fluoridated water, and most US dentists agree that fluoride prevents tooth decay. In 1999, the Center for Disease Control (CDC) named the fluoridation of community water one of the top 10 public health achievements of the 20th century. Fluoride strengthens tooth enamel, and it allows teeth damaged by acid to repair, or remineralize, themselves.

Mass Medication

Fluoridation of our water in the US started January 12, 1945 in Grand Rapids, Michigan. Back then asbestos lined our pipes, lead was in our gasoline, PCBs filled our transformers and DDT was deemed so "safe and effective" that officials felt no qualms spraying kids in school classrooms and seated at picnic tables. One by one all these chemicals have been banned except fluoridation! Did you know that western Europe allows individuals the right to choose, or refuse, fluoride. While water fluoridation is often credited with causing the reduction in tooth decay that has occurred in the US over the past 50 years, the same reductions in tooth decay have occurred in all western countries, most of which have never added fluoride to their water. Comprehensive data from the World Health Organization shows that tooth decay rates are just as low as rates in the US.

Too Much Fluoride?

In 2006, a panel of dentists, toxicologists, and epidemiologists assembled by the National Research Council (NRC) determined that the level of fluoride allowed in community drinking water in this country is too high. More is better–right? The State of California Department of Public Health has stated: *"Increases in fluoride concentration in excess of 1 part per million (ppm) do not further decrease the occurrence of dental caries but do increase the risk of objectionable fluorosis* (mottling of the teeth)." It is usually accepted by medical authorities that children should have no more than 1 mg/day, and adults, 1.5 to 2 mg/day. However according to Dr. Albert Burgstahler, University of Kansas, the average adult daily intake today is 2 to 3 mg. Two liters of water alone used in drinking and cooking will contain your total "safe" dose for the day. Why does the toothpaste label state, *"Keep out of reach of children under 6 years of age. If more than is used for brushing is accidentally swallowed, get medical help or contact a Poison Control Center right away."?* Because fluoride can be a neurotoxin and potentially tumorigenic if swallowed. 50% of the fluoride we swallow each day accumulates in our bones.

Fluoride Toxicity?

Did you know that in addition to the fluoride ingested in water, fluoride is also contained in plastics, pharmaceuticals/anesthetics (medicines), cigarettes, and many foods; such as fruit juices, soda, black and green teas, beer, some wines, mechanically deboned chicken, meat, fish/ sea food, gelatin (stored in animal fat), some processed foods/cereals, insecticides on fruits and vegetables, and fluoridated toothpaste (200 mg. in a 50 g. tube). Tea drinking by itself can cause low level fluoride poisoning and possibly arthritis if done to excess! Fluoride compounds are highly persistent, fat soluble and accumulate in the planet's food chains and our body fat to toxic levels over the years. It is suggested that up to 66% of fluoride taken into our bodies comes from bathing and clothes washed in fluoridated water.

The Chemistry Of Fluoride

Fluoride is a halogen, like chlorine, bromide and iodine. It is the smallest and most reactive element in the halogen family (elements with 7 electrons in their outer shell). Fluorine exists as a gas, but in nature it is attached to other elements as the negatively charged ion fluoride, most notably to hydrogen, calcium, sodium, aluminum, sulfur, and silicon. Sodium fluoride, a by-product of aluminum smelting, initially was used to fluoridate water. Silicofluorides (fluoride combined with silicon), wastes of phosphate fertilizer production, are now used almost exclusively for fluoridation. Fluorine is also present in compounds called organofluorines, where fluorine atoms (not fluoride anions) are tightly bound to carbon. Teflon (poly-tetra-fluoro-ethylene)-safe to 500°, Gore-Tex, and many drugs, Prozac (fluoxetine) and Cipro (ciprofloxacin).

Water Fluoridation

The chemicals that have been most commonly used for artificial water fluoridation include:

1. Sodium fluoride (NaF) - widespread use is in toothpaste and other dental treatments. This compound in high levels is a highly toxic

protoplasmic poison which accumulates in the body.

2. Hydrofluorosilicic acid (H_2SiF_6) - a liquid compound that has been used for artificial water fluoridation in Canada for over 60 years. This chemical was chosen because of its low cost and widespread availability (as a waste product from chemical processing of phosphate rock: especially for separation of uranium from other ores, aluminum, steel, ceramics and phosphate fertilizers).

3. Sodium silicofluoride (Na_2SiF_6) - a solid compound related to hydrofluorosilicic acid. This form of fluoride is used in high concentrations to kill rats and crop-eating insects. Silicofluorides ((H_2SiF_6) & Na_2SiF_6)) are classified as Hazardous Waste according to the Basel Convention, Environment Canada and United States Environmental Protection Agency (US EPA).

Sodium Vs Calcium Fluoride

Municipal employees who add fluoridation chemicals to public water systems must wear protective clothing and respirators. Industrial workers regularly exposed to fluorine, the gas form of fluoride, have suffered skin, lung, and gastrointestinal problems; it has even been fatal for some. Fluoride is usually added to soft water from our cities, but fluorides occurring in nature, usually in the form of calcium fluoride, are found in hard water containing high levels of calcium and magnesium. Physiologically, the body copes better with the effects of fluoride if calcium and magnesium are present, and in cases of chronic and acute fluoride poisoning, the antidote is calcium. Sodium fluoride is highly soluble in water, whereas calcium fluoride is only slightly soluble. Calcium fluoride is 85 times less toxic than sodium fluoride. Sodium fluoride is more toxic than lead and slightly less toxic than arsenic.

Fluoride Is For Children

97% of western Europe (Austria, Belgium, Denmark, Finland, France, Germany, Iceland, Italy, Luxembourg, Netherlands, Northern Ireland, Norway, Scotland, Sweden, and Switzerland) do not have water fluoridation, but has been as equally successful as the US, if not more so, in tackling tooth decay. If fluoride was necessary for strong teeth, you would expect to find it in breast milk, but the level there is 0.01 ppm, which is 100 times LESS than in fluoridated tap water *(IOM, 1997)*. Children in non-fluoridated communities are already getting the so-called "optimal" doses from other sources *(Heller et al, 1997)*, with most already being over-exposed to fluoride. Doses of fluoride at 0.4 to 0.8 ppm can cause mottling of the teeth in children by damaging the enamel (dental fluorosis) of a high percentage of children. Between 30 and 50% of children have dental fluorosis on at least two teeth in optimally fluoridated communities *(Heller et al, 1997 and McDonagh et al, 2000)*. Major dental researchers also concede that fluoride is ineffective at preventing pit and fissure tooth decay, which is the cause of 85% of the tooth decay experienced by children (JADA 1984; Gray 1987; White 1993; Pinkham 1999). The largest survey conducted in the US showed only a minute difference in tooth decay between children who had lived all their lives in fluoridated compared to non-fluoridated communities. The difference was not clinically significant nor shown to be statistically significant *(Brunelle & Carlos, 1990)*. The worst tooth decay in the United States occurs in the poor neighborhoods of our largest cities, the vast majority of which have been fluoridated for decades. When fluoridation has been halted in communities in Finland, former East Germany, Cuba and Canada, tooth decay did not go up but continued to go down *(Maupome et al, 2001; Kunzel and Fischer, 1997, 2000; Kunzel et al, 2000 and Seppa et al, 2000)*.

Dementia, IQ And Fluoride

The National Research Council (NRC) states that fluoride can damage the brain. Animal studies conducted in the 1990s by Environmental Protection Agency (EPA) scientists found dementia-like effects at the same concentration (1 ppm) used to fluoridate water, while human studies have found adverse effects on IQ at levels as low as 0.9 ppm among children with nutrient deficiencies, and levels of 1.8 ppm among children with adequate nutrient intake. In 1942, Nazi Germany became the world's largest producer of aluminum (and Sodium Fluoride). Fluoride was used in the concentration camps to render the prisoners docile and inhibit their questioning of authority. Russia added fluoride to the water in its concentration camps as well during this time. In 2005, Chinese children drinking well water with very high levels of fluoride scored poorly on intelligence testing compared to those with lower exposures.

Lead Toxicity Increased From Fluoride Exposure

In human studies, the fluoridating agents most commonly used in the US not only increased the uptake of lead into children's blood (Masters and Coplan, 1999, 2000), but were also associated with an increase in violent behavior. Lead interferes with the neurotransmitter dopamine, which controls impulsive and violent behavior; and studies show that lead pollution is linked to higher rates of violent crime. The average violent crime rate in US counties that have lead pollution is 56 percent higher when their drinking water is fluoridated. (Fluoride 2005;38:1-5, 11-22).

Mood And Sleep Disorders

Fluoride accumulates in our pineal gland more than any other body organ, possibly lowering the production of melatonin and serotonin, very important regulatory hormones (Luke, 1997, 2001). Therefore, fluoride could cause sleep and mood disorders. Did you know that day time exercise and meditation/prayer increases melatonin production. Also noted in these studies is an acceleration of puberty in females.

Thyroid Dysfunction And Obesity

The NRC states that fluoride is an endocrine disrupter and has warned that doses of fluoride (0.01-0.03 mg/kg/day) achievable by drinking fluoridated water, may reduce the function of the thyroid among individuals with low-iodine intake. Up until the 1970s, European doctors used fluoride as a thyroid-suppressing medication for patients with HYPER-thyroidism (over-active thyroid). Fluoride was utilized because it was found to be effective at reducing the activity of the thyroid gland - even at doses as low as 2 mg/day. Fluoride contributes to hypothyroidism by binding to the thyroid receptors instead of iodine. Low thyroid levels can lead to loss of mental acuity (brain fog), being cold all the time, depression, dry skin and weight gain/obesity.

Aluminum And Fluoride

In animal studies, fluoride at 1 ppm in drinking water increases the uptake of aluminum into the brain (Varner et al, 1998). Cooking in aluminum cookware with water containing fluorides increases the aluminum concentration by up to a thousand times more than cooking in fluorine-free water. This could increase the possibility of aluminum induced Alzheimer disease.

Infertility

Counties with 3 ppm or more of fluoride in their water have lower fertility rates in both males and females (Freni, 1994). The margin of safety between the so-called therapeutic benefit of reducing dental decay and causing harm is either nonexistent or precariously low.

Cancer

Fluoride at 1 ppm shows increased tumor growth rate in the lab and impairment of DNA to repair itself. Fluoride disrupts hydrogen bonds. Hydrogen bonds are the velcro strips that hold the enzyme in our bodies in a certain shape. Increased cancer death rates are seen by fluoride destroying over 100 body enzymes, interfering with mineral and vitamin functions in your body system. Enzymes trigger specific reactions in the body and are long-chain proteins held in certain shapes. They act like a key in a lock. Fluoride changes the shape of the enzymes so that they no longer fit. Since enzymes are proteins, once they've been changed, they're now foreign-looking. The body now treats them as invaders, even though they're part of your body. This is known as an autoimmune situation - the body attacks itself. Fluoride comes along and hydrolyzes the enzyme: cuts the velcro strips away. The shape collapses. No more enzyme; now just a foreign protein that your body attacks. With constant inflammation attacking the body cells, they mutate and can become cancer cells.

Fluoride In Bones

Fluoride at 1 ppm interferes with collagen metabolism and bone formation. Fluoride accumulates in our bones and makes them more brittle over time. Scientists at EPA report drinking fluorinated water has been directly linked in adults to bone de-mineralization, carpal-tunnel syndrome, and arthritis by interfering with calcium deposits. July 9, 1998, the Manchester Guardian reported news of fluoride poisoned water in Central India, from untested wells drilled in the 1980s, causing severe arthritic damage to tens of millions of people. A lifetime exposure to fluoride contributes to higher rates of hip fracture in the elderly with levels as low 1.5 ppm daily. There are serious, but yet unproven, concerns about a connection between fluoridation and osteosarcoma in young men *(Cohn, 1992)*. Up to half of adolescents who develop osteosarcoma die within a few years of their diagnosis. Mutations in the p53 gene are the most commonly observed genetic alterations in human cancer. The NRC concludes that fluoride probably causes mutations in p53 which cause osteosarcomas.

Fluoride Ingestion

The benefits of fluoride are clearly topical, not systemic (CDC, 1999, 2001), so fluoridated toothpaste, which is universally available, is a more rational approach to delivering fluoride to the target organ (teeth) while minimizing exposure to the rest of us.

So What Can I Do?

- Pray without ceasing.
- Do not drink bottled water/sports drinks, soda or fruit/vegetable juices (usually made from fluoridated water), you may drink you own juiced fruits or vegetables.
- Adults, do not use fluoridated toothpaste or mouthwashes.
- Do not drink teas.
- Increase your plant based calcium/magnesium in your diet.

• Make sure you are getting enough vitamin D (essential for calcium adsorption).

- Avoid animal products, because fluoride collects in their fat.
- Check your water filter for its ability to remove fluoride. The fluoride anion diameter size is 0.64 nm which is smaller than the usual filter pore size. Boiling or carbon filters will eliminate all traces of chlorine from city water, but will not eliminate fluoride, which is only eliminated by distilling your water or using a reverse osmosis filter. Distilled water tends to be acidic with a pH of 5.5 and lacks trace minerals. Distilling your water is not suggested for long term use (years).
- 1000 mg. per day of magnesium, preferably in a highly absorbable form, such as magnesium lactate, malate or gluconate and/or 6 almonds a day. Avoid magnesium aspartate as aspartic acid is an excitatory amino acid.
- 2000 mg. of calcium citrate daily. Avoid calcium from living creatures, such as animal bone, coral or oyster shells. They may contain toxic lead, cadmium and arsenic.
- Take 2000 IU of vitamin D daily. Experiments show protection for embryos of pregnant animals exposed to fluoride.
- Take 2000 mg (minimum) of vitamin C daily.
- Iodine supplementation has been clinically demonstrated to increase the urine excretion of sodium fluoride from the body as calcium fluoride. I use 'Iodoral' brand, 50 mg. a day for one month, then 12.5 a day thereafter.
- Lecithin two tablespoons of granules a day is recommended as an adjunct to using iodine for excreting fluorides.
- Boron 3 mg. a day has been studied around the world with pronounced success for fluoride detoxification.
- Dry Saunas combined with exercise releases sodium fluoride stored in fatty tissues. It can be intense enough to cause side effects or an occasional healing crisis. So keep the pure water intake high and drink some chickweed tea to protect the kidneys while using a highly absorbable cal/mag supplement.
- Cilantro pesto with chlorella (algae) chelates heavy metals, including fluoride salts (sodium fluoride). 400 mg. of cilantro a day can markedly improve your heavy metals load in your body in just 2 weeks.

References:

Featherstone JDB. (2000). *The Science and Practice of Caries Prevention. Journal of the American Dental Association.* 131: 887-899. (Additional references available at: www.fluoridealert.org/health/teeth/caries/topical-systemic.html)

Centers for Disease Control and Prevention (2001). Recommendations for Using Fluoride to Prevent and Control Dental Caries in the United States. Mortality and Morbidity Weekly Review. (MMWR). August 17. 50(RR14):1-42.

Grandjean P, Landrigan P. (2006). *Developmental neurotoxicity of industrial chemicals.* The Lancet, November 8.

National Research Council. (2006). *Fluoride in Drinking Water: A Scientific Review of EPA's Standards.* National Academies Press, Washington D.C. p. 173-188.

Varner JA, et al. (1998). *Chronic Administration of Aluminum-Fluoride and Sodium-Fluoride to Rats in Drinking Water: Alterations in Neuronal and Cerebrovascular Integrity.* Brain Research. 784: 284-298.

Lin Fa-Fu, et al. (1991). *The relationship of a low-iodine and high-fluoride environment to subclinical cretinism in Xinjiang.* Iodine Deficiency Disorder Newsletter. Vol. 7. No. 3.
Xiang Q, et al. (2003a). Effect of fluoride in drinking water on children's intelligence. Fluoride 36: 84-94; 198-199.

National Toxicology Program. (1990). *Toxicology and Carcinogenesis Studies of Sodium Fluoride in F344/N Rats and B6C3f1 Mice.* Technical report Series No. 393. NIH Publ. No 91-2848. National Institute of Environmental Health Sciences, Research Triangle Park, N.C.

Hoover RN, et al. (1991). *Time trends for bone and joint cancers and osteosarcomas in the Surveillance, Epidemiology and End Results (SEER) Program.* National Cancer Institute In: Review of Fluoride: Benefits and Risks. US Public Health Service. Appendix E & F.

Cohn PD. (1992). *A Brief Report On The Association Of Drinking Water Fluoridation And The Incidence of Osteosarcoma Among Young Males.* New Jersey Department of Health Environ. Health Service: 1- 17.

Bassin EB, Wypij D, Davis RB, Mittleman MA. (2006). *Age-specific Fluoride Exposure in Drinking Water and Osteosarcoma (United States).* Cancer Causes and Control 17: 421-8.

Johnson W, et al. (1979). *Fluoridation and bone disease in renal patients.* In: E Johansen, DR Taves, TO Olsen, Eds. Continuing Evaluation of the Use of Fluorides. AAAS Selected Symposium. Westview Press, Boulder, Colorado. pp. 275-293.

Ittel TH, et al. (1992). *Effect of fluoride on aluminum-induced bone disease in rats with renal failure.* Kidney International 41: 1340-1348.

Ayoob S, Gupta AK. (2006). *Fluoride in Drinking Water: A Review on the Status and Stress Effects.* Critical Reviews in Environmental Science and Technology 36:433–487
http://www.consumerhealth.org/articles/display.cfm?ID=19990817225011

http://www.prevention.com/health/health/healthy-living/the-danger-in-your-water/article/319972e50d803110VgnVCM10000013281eac____

http://www.fluoridealert.org/health/kidney/

http://www.fluoridealert.org/health/biblio.html

Fluoride Action Network I 802-338-5577 I info@fluoridealert.org

http://www.time.com/time/specials/packages/article/0,28804,1976909_1976895_1976898,00.html#ixzz0qfpy4VdX

Wang SX, ZH Wang, XT Cheng, J Li, ZP Sang, XD Zhang, LL Han, SY Qiao, ZM Wu and ZQ Wang. 2007. *Arsenic and fluoride exposure in drinking water: children's IQ and growth in Shanyin County, Shanxi province, China.* Environmental Health Perspectives 115(4):643-7
Luke J. (2001). Fluoride deposition in the aged human pineal gland. Caries Research 35:125-128

National Research Council. (2006), *Fluoride in Drinking Water: A Scientific Review of EPA's Standards.* National Academies Press, Washington D.C. p 223

Mt. Pleasant, MI will reduce fluoride levels in water to 0.7 ppm commissioners voted June 15, 2010.

http://www.naturalnews.com/026605_fluoride_fluorides_detox.html

http://www.organic-vida.com/community/environmental-news/cilantro-helps-detox-heavy-metals.html Nov. 9, 2009

THE POWER OF ENDORPHINS

- The "Feel Good" Molecules
- Low Levels Cause Depression And Fatigue

Endorphins Work On Morphine/Opiate Receptors

Endorphins are best known to those who exercise a lot, because they cause a sense of euphoria or "Runners High" from their release. Endorphins are polypeptides containing 30 amino acid units that bind to opiate receptors in the brain and can elicit feelings of euphoria, appetite modulation, hormone release and have pain-relieving properties. Endorphins are neurotransmitters that interact with morphine receptor neurons to reduce pain. In chronic pain disorders, endorphins are found in high numbers.

Three Types Of Endorphins

There are three types of endorphins: beta endorphins, found primarily in the pituitary gland of the brain; enkephalins and dynorphins, both distributed through out the nervous system but are mainly located in brain areas. Dynorphin and enkephalin peptides regulate extra pyramidal motor function, cardiovascular and water balance systems, eating, signal processing and pain reception.

Effects Of Endorphins

Endorphins are produced in response to stress/pain (exercise is perceived as stress by the body) and they produce key effects on the body/mind: they enhance the immune system, they relieve pain, tension, anger, confusion and anxiety, they improve appetite control, they reduce stress and they postpone the aging process. Endorphins are released by the anterior pituitary and from lymphocytes directly into inflamed tissue in response to stress and pain. Endorphins are also involved in the regulation of the female menstrual cycle, as well as influencing the response of numerous hormones, including growth hormone, adrenocorticotropin (ACTH), prolactin, catecholamines, cortisol and dihydroepiandrosterone (DHEA).

Do You Have A High Or Low Pain Threshold?

Some people appear to be genetically deficient or don't produce as much endorphin as others. This can make these deficient people more susceptible to pain. Thus, we have people who have high or low pain thresholds, probably from their endorphin production ability.

Exercise And Endorphins

Prolonged exercise raises endorphin levels and trained individuals degrade endorphins more slowly than untrained individuals. This can explain why exercise training can cause a greater tolerance for extended exercise and pain. That's why I say, "You'll rust out before you wear out."

Chronic Pain

Endorphins are known to block pain receptors and are released by immune cells in response to a stressful/painful event. Endorphins become deficient if pain is constant and unrelenting. Endorphins are stored in your adrenal glands. Another reason for chronic pain is that your body may become tolerant to its own endorphins and this may cause pain levels to increase. Taurine, an essential amino acid found in beans and seeds, helps inhibit the development of tolerance to opioid peptides. It is found in most nuts.

During early inflammation/pain (six hours), all three endorphins are activated and block different receptors for the perception of pain. At later stages (four days), pain receptor blockade is produced predominately by beta endorphin, acting at peripheral receptors influencing pain perception.

Sugar And Low Endorphins

Sugar consumption is known to precipitate or worsen major depression. Some researchers believe that a high sugar intake in the diet correlates with low levels of beta endorphins, leading to depression.

Weight And Endorphins

The release of endorphin neuropeptides decreases your appetite via the hypothalamus in your brain. The hormone leptin, which is involved in the regulation of fat intake, is a direct target for endorphin interaction. Beta endorphins are required for the normal regulation of your appetite and satiety. Endorphins are also required for a favorable regulation of your energy use (weight homeostasis).

Depression And Low Levels Of Endorphins

Phenylalanine is an essential amino acid. It is present in bananas, but one of the highest levels is in almonds. D-phenylalanine has an analgesic action and has been shown to be associated with brain chemicals relating to pain sensation. D-phenylalanine is an inhibitor of the endorphin degrading enzyme-enkephalinase; thus increasing the available endorphin to the body. DL-phenylalanine is a mixture of D-phenylalanine and L-phenylalanine. All forms (D, L, DL) are required as an essential amino acid and have been tested in depression with favorable results.

Phenylalanine is a building block for various proteins and the Lform is used in the production of neurotransmitters such as L-dopa (aspartame can be a neuro toxin blocking these neurotransmitters, so avoid NutraSweet® and Equal®); epinephrine, norepinephrine and the making of phenylethylamine, a naturally occurring substance in the brain that causes mood elevation. The D-form has been found to help stabilize Parkinsonism.

Amino Acids And Endorphin Production

Endorphins are formed mainly from the essential amino acid protein tyrosine. Tyrosine is found in bananas, avocado, seeds, and beans. Tyrosine serves as a precursor also of epinephrine, thyroxine and melanin. Insulin causes active transport of many of the amino acids into the cells. Among the essential amino acids most strongly transported by insulin and growth hormone are valine, leucine, isoleucine, tyrosine andphenylalanine. So to get insulin to work properly, we need to exercise. Thus exercising increases the endorphin release and the absorption of the essential amino acids into the body, which increases endorphins.

Memory And Endorphins

Those with higher endorphin levels learned better and remembered what they have learned longer.

How To Stimulate Your Endorphin Production

So why have I told you all this? Because of the simple God-given ways to feel better and improve your life on this earth! So what stimulates endorphins? Exercise, nutrition, sunshine, uplifting music, massage and chiropractic, acupuncture, local electrical stimulation (TENS unit), hydrotherapy (including hot and cold fominations, Jacuzzi, daily baths and sauna use) and meditation/prayer.

References:

Davis, *"Endorphins: New Waves In Brain Chemistry."* Garden Press, New York Dial Press, 1984.

McArdle, W.D., *"Exercise Physiology: Energy, Nutrition and Human Performance,"* 2004.

Beckmann, H., *"DL-phenylalanine vs. Imipramine: A Double Blind Controlled Study,"* Arch Psych Nervenkr 1979 Jul 4;227 (1):49-58.

Nutri-Notes, *"Endorphins,"* 2005 May; Vol.9, #5:1-9.

Sabelli, H.C., *"Clinical Studies On The Phenylethylamine Hypothesis Of Affective Disorder: Urine And Blood Phenylacetic Acid And Phenylalanine Dietary Supplements,"* J. Clin Psych 1986;47:660-70.

Fischer, E. *"Therapy Of Depression By Phenylalanine,"* Arzneimittelforschung, 1975;25:132.

Westover, A.N., *"A Cross-national Relationship Between Sugar Consumption And Major Depression?"* Depress Anxiety, 2002;16(3):118-120.

Machelska, H., *"Intrinsic Pain Inhibition,"* J Neuroimmunol, 2003 Aug;14(1-2):30-39.

Appleyard, S.M., *"A Role For The Endogenous Opioid Beta-endorphin In Energy Homeostasis,"* Endocrinolgy, 2003 May;144(5):1753-1760.

Jin, X., *"Influence Of Beta-endorphin On Function Of Immune SystemOf Patients With Cerebral Hemorrhage,"* Zhonghua Yi Xue Za Zhi, 2003 Aug 25;83(16):1409-1412.

FIBROMYALGIA SYNDROME

- The Metabolic Work Up
- Remember** What Helps One Person May Not Benefit The Next.

The American College of Rheumatology in 1992 established two criteria for a diagnosis of fibromyalgia:

1) Pain in all four quadrants of the body and in the axial skeleton (bones of the head, throat, chest and spine) that's been present on a more-or-less continuous basis for at least three months.

2) Pain in at least 11 of 18 tender points, which are specific spots on the body that hurt when pressure is applied.

If you have different symptoms (and most people with the diagnosis of fibromyalgia do), then you do not have fibromyalgia. But what do you have??? It is important to make sure you do not have: Rheumatoidarthritis, Multiple sclerosis, Lupus, Lyme's disease, Myasthenia gravis, Crohn's disease, auto-immune disorders, HIV, etc.

1. **Heavy Metal Toxicity**

Note Doctor's Data – (HCPCS#'s) Urine toxic element Mercury (985.0), Arsenic (961.2) and Lead (984.1) Screening blood or urine Testing: Great Smokies LAB: 253-0621 (Urine 24 hour $55.00) Nash,D., "Blood Lead, Blood Pressure, and Hypertension In Perimenopausal and Postmenopausal Women," JAMA 2–3;289:1523-32.Treatment: John Wilson M.D. Great Smokies Medical Center for Chelation, 828/252-9833 James Biddle M.D. Asheville Integrative Medicine for Chelation, 828/252-5545

2. **Food Allergies**

Wheat/Celiac Sprue intolerances. Check AntiGliadin Antibodies if diarrhea present. Testing: Rast Blood Test. May include Drugs (995.2), grasses (477.8), animals (477.8), molds (477.8), herbs (693.1) or specific foods.

Soy product intolerances can cause fatigue, headaches, rashes, stomach and chest pain. Treatment: Elimination trials

3. **Multiple Chemical Sensitivity Syndrome**

Chemical/Environmental Sensitivities; respiratory fumes/vapors (506.9). Formaldehyde, perfumes, cleaners, etc. Treatment: Elimination trials

4. **Clotting Abnormalities**

A positive D-Dimer blood test because of inappropriate fibrous stranding may require heparin, lovonex or coumadin treatment. Acquired coagulation defect (286.7), Thyroid peroxidase antibodies, Lupus anti-coagulant, Anti-phospholipid antibodies, Factor 5 Ligand deficiency, etc. Empiric Trial for Headaches that transiently respond to diuretics or prednisone and clotting abnormalities.

5. **Endocrine Insufficiency**

Pituitary and other endocrine abnormalities are far more common than generally realized. Evaluate fully, including growth hormone levels (Insulin Growth Factor 1-IGF-1). Measure free T3 and free T4 levels with TSH and check basal AM body temperatures. Test for auto-antibodies. Thyroid abnormalities require Cytomel 5 mcg up to 50 mcg BID or Amour Thyroid 30 mg (T3 and T4 animal extract supplies both T3/T4 in one pill). Clinical hypothyroidism can result from receptor blockade and the inability to convert T4 to the active hormone T3 (converts to reverse T3 instead), thus hypothyroidism can exist despite normal serum hormone levels. Treatment: push T3 and T4 to high normal range. Consider sustained release T3: 45-120 mcg a day. Hypofunction pituitary (253.1); Anterior Pituitary Deficiency (253.4) evaluation to include ACTH, LH, FSH, Prolactin, IGF-1, Cortisol and TSH blood levels.

6. **Narcolepsy Symptoms** (347.0)

Falling asleep during the day can be treated with amphetamines. Treatment: Provigil 200 mg BID or other similar med (there areseveral). Ritalin in adults may help too.

7. **Sleep Disorders**

Most fatigued patients don't sleep. Sleep Disorders may require a work-up for oxygen and/or CPAP. Apnea sleep disturbance (780.51) or Obstructive Sleep Apnea. Start with a 24 hour O_2 sat. study-Free with doctor's prescription. Sleep Centers at local hospitals and any Durable Medical Equipment (DME) company that supplies O_2.

8. **Fat Malabsorption Syndrome**

BodyBio Fatty Acid Test (In depth Supportive Red Cell Lipid Analysis)-Great Smokies Lab 828 253-0621 If there is any suggestion of autism, this study is essential. Treatment as outlined by deficiencies.

9. **Muscle Aching**

Primary Myopathy (359.89) Not all of these may help, but a trial of one at a time may.

A. Creatine Monohydrate makes more calcium available to your muscles and boosts water levels inside your muscle cells, which helps them synthesize proteins and store glycogen. Caffeine negates this good effect. Check Creatine level. Supplement up to 5 grams a day (found in health food stores in weight lifting section).

B. MSM (Methylsufonylmethane) Sulfur compounds are needed for bones, teeth, collagen (the protein in connective tissue) and a healthy immune response to inflammation. Sulfur is needed for the manufacture of many proteins including muscles. 6 grams a day in divided doses.

C. Nitroglycerin .3 mg ½ to ¼ tab sublingual for muscle pain relief. If there is no improvement consider this patient to have a sulfur insufficiency. Treat with MSM 2000 mg and up.

D. B12 increases the synaptic relay between nerve cell ends and thus clinically improving muscle/ nerve weakness. Sublingual or nasal OTC, 1000 mcg to 5000 mcg every day.

E. Co Enzyme Q10 supports the energy producing pathways in the mitochondria (tiny cell power houses). 100 mg to 400 mg a day.

F. NADH is a co-enyzme needed in the production of ATP (the cells packets of energy). 1000 mg to 5000 mg a day 30 minutes before breakfast.

G. B complex including B6 (stress tab formula), one each day.

H. Trial of treatment as if patient had Lyme's Disease-Cat's Claw (nature's Cipro), 5 drops twice a day.

10. **Nitric Oxide Deficiency**

If Nitroglycerin (NTG 1/150 sl) has given you some temporary muscle ache relief, try adding L Arginine. NTG and L-Arginine stimulate production and release of nitric oxide from the endothelial vessel lining. L-Arginine helps sustains nitric oxide levels in the human body and stimulates the release of growth hormone from the pituitary gland (when blood sugar levels are not high). When you move or exercise, your body naturally releases nitric oxide, which affects the endothelial dilating pathway. Nitric oxide is the muscles "cell signaling" molecule that activities protein synthesis (the process of making new muscle out of protein). Nitric oxide enhances insulin sensitivity, which helps to boost creatine absorption into your muscle cells without the use of sugar. Treatment: L-Arginine (nitric oxide precursor) 8 grams to 14 grams a day Amino Acid Deficiency (270.9) Hambrecht, R., "Correction of Endothelial Dysfunction in Chronic Heart Failure: Additional Effects of Exercise Training and Oral L-Arginine Supplementation," J Am Coll Cardiol 2000;35:706-713.

11. **Dehydroepiandrosterone Sulfate (DHEA) Deficiency**

Called the "Fountain of Youth Hormone," "The Master Hormone" and the "Mother Hormone," DHEA assists in the product of vital hormones. It is the precursor chemical ring that makes up your body's steroids, estrogen, testosterone, cholesterol and vitamin D hormones. Endocrine deficiency; Adrenal gland hypofunction (564.1) Lab: DHEA-S level. Treatment:

If level is 50 to 200 mg/dl, start DHEA at 25mg a day. If the level is less than 50 mg/dl, start DHEA at 50 mg day. Titrate to normalize the laboratory blood level.

12. **Irritable Bowel Disorder (IBS)**

Keep a food intake diary to evaluate for food sensitivities as triggers of IBS symptoms. Treatment: Food avoidance, particularly lactose and complex food combinations. Melatonin 10 mg a day. This dose may help sleep too.

13. **Viral Overload**

Transfer Factor has some success in treating symptoms of Cytomegalovirus-CMV (078.5), Human Herpes Virus 6-HHV6 A&B and Epstein Barr Virus (acute-075.0; chronic 139.8). Transfer factor has been shown to neutralizes Candida Albicans overgrowth and suppress Chlamydia. Transfer Factor is extracted from cow's first milk (may be derived from chicken sources as well). Colostrum's sole purpose is to transfer immunity from mother to the baby's immature immune system. Transfer Factor stabilizes autoimmune dysfunction by helping to eliminate "immune cross talk" and reestablishes immune balance. Treatment: Don't treat with just Colostrum. Transfer Factor has different formulas. Transfer Factor: 200 mg to 1000 mg a day. Keep cold and take on an empty stomach.

14. **Syncope/Fainting**

Neurally Mediated Hypotension-NMH (458.0) can be diagnosed by Tilt Table Testing. Treatment can dramatically lessen fatigue, palpitations, wooziness and increase stamina by allowing the brainstem to talk to the spinal column, by restoring the Adrenaline "Fright or Flight" mechanism. Also symptoms of Postural Orthostatic Tachycardia Syndrome (POTS) and Parkinsonism sometimes respond to the same treatments. Treatment for symptomatic autonomic failure:

A. Suboccipital Decompression (neck/skull surgery) resolves/lessens symptoms in 85% of patients.

B. If hypovolemia is the cause of a positive tilt table test then increase sodium (Salt) intake and fluid intake, TED hose and eat smaller-more frequent meals. One may add Florinef (fludrocortisone) .1 mg BID plus potassium or ProAmitine(midodrine) starting at 2.5 mg three times a day and increasing stepwise. Other choices may include: ephedrine, sudafed and dexadrine, Sandostatin (octreotide) 150-750 mcg subq in divided doses 2-4 times a day, erythropoietin (procrit), and indomethacin 50 mg three times a day.

C. If there is reproduction of symptoms with tachycardia and inappropriate hypotension during isuprel or dobutamin estimulation during the tilt table test adding a beta blocker may help. Serotonin agonist have helped rarely.

15. **Magnesium Deficiency**

Magnesium deficiency (275.2) is very often present in people with fatigue and quite severe. Hyper-reflexa, muscle twitches, myocardial irritability, poor stamina and recurrent muscle spasms are clues that the patient may have an intracellular magnesium deficiency. 99% of the body's magnesium is inside the cells, so blood testing is inadequate.
1 gm IV or IM at least once a week until neuromuscular irritability has cleared, then oral maintenance of one Tbsp black strap Molasses/day or liquid magnesium/calcium source for at least 1000 mg a day. Once stable, add a calcium/magnesium/vitamin D tab 2-4 a day. Avoid magnesium if you have diarrhea or renal failure. Avoid molasses if you are a diabetic. Combination magnesium and malic acid (Krebs energy cycle) also helps in some cases more than just magnesium alone (trade name-Super Malic 3-6 tabs/day).

16. **Candida Overgrowth**

Yeast overgrowth causes fatigue symptoms. Yeast thrives in an acidic environment. Jump start your body's change to higher alkalinity with juicing fresh veggies (cabbage works well for several of my patients). Avoid sugars, fried foods, sodas, caffeine products, McDonald's type diet, alcohol, and combinations that can cause fermentation in the gut (milk and sugar). All of these foods are extremely acidic and promote yeast overgrowth. Treatment: Diet change to more natural/fresh/raw.

17. **Vitamin D Deficiency**

Vitamin D deficiency (82306) is very common and when corrected can markedly improve fatigue symptoms. Blood test for 25 Hydroxy (25OHD3) deficiency. OTC Vitamin D 5,000 units a day. Prescription: 50,000 units weekly.

18. **My Recommendations For All Of My Tired Patients**

My "fibromyalgia" patients all do better with liquid trace minerals, including extra magnesium (269.3), B12 500-2000 units sl/day OTC (281.0), 1 oz/kg of water/day, vitamin D 5,000 unit a day and omega-3 (Flax seed/Fish Oil) supplement 4 grams/day.

OTC=Over The Counter
(###) are CPT codes for your physician.

OVER THE COUNTER TREATMENTS FOR INFLAMMATORY BOWEL DISEASE

- Crohn's Disease

Crohn's disease is caused by inflammation (the body is attacking itself-auto-immune), sores and ulcerations of the bowel cause scaring, especially of the ileum (the last portion of the small bowel). One in every 1000 people in western countries have this disease. Some researchers, including me, believe Crohn's disease is from a form of tuberculosis called MAP (Mycobacterium Avium Para-tuberculosis). We all agree that what ever causes Crohn's disease has to be a combination of both genetic and environmental factors that give rise to this gut problem. Whatever it is, everyone in western society is exposed to it equally, but only those predisposed genetically get the disease (runs in families, communities, etc).

Crohn's disease is a hyper-immune state with too many helper T cells and not enough balance of suppressor T cells. Therefore, I've found that herbs that increase the immune response, like Echinacea, make me worse. There are three regions on the chromosomes that have been identified (12, 14, 16) as containing faulty genes contributing to Crohn's disease. Scientists believe there are at least six chromosomes involved. People with one copy of the defective gene, which alters the immune system's response to bacteria and food in the gut, have twice the normal risk of developing Crohn's disease, while those with two copies of the gene have 15 to 20 times the risk and so on.

One of the cytokines that is abnormality high in Crohn's disease (pro-inflammatory-causes inflammation) is Tumor Necrosis Factor-Alpha (TNF-α). This can be down regulated to normal levels and can cause remission in Crohn's disease patients.*

The following treatment options will not effect an acute flare of disease, this will requirement prescription help; but, these options may help keep you in a longer remission between flares. Consult your Health Care Provider with any of these therapies.

All suggestions I have found in the medical literature. I have tried all of these at one time or another. One thing I've found is that all Crohn's disease patients respond differently to treatments. Here are a few to try, but not all at once please.

- Omega-3 (sources include: fish oil, borage oil, primrose oil and flax seed) Requires 3-4 months for effect. Omega-3 normalizes TNF-α and COX-2 pathways.* Grind fresh two tablespoons of flax seed a day (best source).

• Avoid dehydration-drink plenty of water. Minimum ounces of water required each day should be: your weight in pounds, divided by 2.2 = ounces of water needed/day.

• Avoid milk products. All Crohn's patients are lactose intolerant. Milk is the carrier for para-tuberculosis, if this is the cause of Crohn's. Some scientists suggest that exposure to the measles virus during pregnancy may be the cause of the faulty DNA/genes.

• Sublingual (under the tongue) vitamin B_{12} 500 mcg weekly or daily during a flare.

• Stinging Nettle leaf 1000 mg a day, contains trace minerals and has an astringent property that cuts down on secretions like blood and mucous.

• Transfer Factor 500 mg a day. This can be found in colostrum (cow's first milk). Yes, you do risk Mad Cow Disease in a couple of years, but my philosophy is you need to feel good now, for you may not be here in a couple of years.*

• Vitamin C two grams (2000 mg) a day; more during a flare. I believe fistulas (draining tracts) are primarily from Vitamin C deficiencies. I've closed my fistulas with large daily doses.

• Vitamin K 10 mg a day. Vitamin K prevents bleeding and acts as an anti-inflammatory. Don't take if you are on coumadin/warfarin.

• Vitamin D 2000 IU a day. Acts as a anti-inflammatory and helps thin bones. Best taken with calcium/magnesium 2:1 ratio (ie, Caltrate with D). Most Crohn's patients have thin bones from malnutrition and steroid treatments. Sun exposure, to as much skin exposed as possible, of 45 minutes minimum, a day, (even sun through a window) can produce up to 10,000 IU of vitamin D.

• Smoking worsens Crohn's disease.

• Barley Green/Wheat Grass etc. (Vitamin K and minerals) daily vs juicing fresh veggies daily. Juicing adds an extra H+ ion to neutralize toxins in your body.

• Activated charcoal for bad gas/diarrhea. Don't use this regularly, because this absorbs the good (medicines/nutrients etc.) and the bad.

• For yeast overgrowth, eat a med-large clove of raw garlic, minced, with a large glass of distilled water 30 minutes before each meal (three times a day for a week).

• Probiotics (lactobacillus acidophilus). Probiotics help stabilize the good bacteria in your bowels and helps resolve bad breath and decreases gas. If you have very smelling stools or changing smell of your stools, this may help the sometimes wild bacterial overgrowth of unwanted bacteria in the intestines. Acidophilus or like product and digestive enzymes each day.

- Turmeric powder 1-3 capsules (300 mg) three times a day for inflammation. Many people cannot take turmeric because it is too spicy and upsets the stomach. Turmeric blocks the inflammation pathway through COX-2, thus blocking TNF-α.*
- Melatonin up to 10 mg a day for short periods of time has been shown to help irritable bowels.
- Peppermint Essential Oil can block smooth muscle abdominal cramping. One drop in a cup of warm water up to four times a day or as needed. Does come in capsules too. This can worsen acid reflux!
- Caraway Oil relaxes the gut wall and thus reduces diarrhea. One drop with water three to four times a day or as needed. Phytotherapy Research, 2000;14:20-23.
- During Crohn's flares 1-2 grams of glutamine (amino acid) fuels the nutrition of the intestinal lining, three times a day. Max six grams a day. Found in the weight lifting section of the Health Food Store. Am J Clin Nutrition 2002;75:789-808. Note: If you are healthy, glutamine has been shown to act as an excitotoxin in the brain.
- Chamomile tea has anti-inflammatory, anti-bacterial and anti-spasm properties, one cup three times a day as needed.
- Slippery Elm Bark can reduce spasms. 400 mg three times day or as needed.
- Aloe Vera juice six ounces three times a day helps soothe bowel inflammation. Aloe promotes healing of the intestinal lining via bradykininase and relaxes the capillaries for increased blood flow and healing.
- Boswellia Serrata (Indian Frankincense) 300 mg three times a day.* Boswellia's acids inhibit a key enzyme involved in the formation of TNF-α.
- Growth Hormone precursors-spray under your tongue as described on the bottle.* NEJM 2000;342(22):1633-1637.
- Liquid trace minerals daily. Crohn's patients are notorious for having zinc and trace mineral deficiencies.
- A heating pad to the abdomen helps reduce spasm pain.
- Two Coconut Macaroon cookies (Archway) has decreased diarrhea from all causes in many patients. I believe the reason is the Propylene Glycol in the cookies.

• DHEA (dehydroepiandrosterone) 25 to 100 mg a day (from Mexican Yams) is a precursor to many of our hormones (including cortisol-prescribed as prednisone). Have your blood level checked (DHEA-S) and take to keep your levels high normal.*

No other disease responds as well as Crohn's to nutritional and alternative therapies.

* lowers (down regulates) high levels of TNF-α.

NEJM 1999;340:253 states that down regulation of TNF-α puts Crohn's disease in remission.

Prescriptions that down regulate TNF-α to more normal levels include: Steroids, Trental, Statins, ACE/ARBs, Amiodarone, Coreg and Plavix.

Prescription drugs that bring TNF-α to zero levels: Remicade (Infliximab) and Thalidomide. I would reserve this treatment only if you are about to die.

By Crohn's patient, Royce K. Bailey, M.D., M.P.H.

GET THE LEAD OUT
- Nature's Chelators

Mercury Toxicity

Recently, the CDC has discussed lowering the toxic blood level of mercury in adults to 10ug/dL from 20ug/dL. Is any mercury OK??? Where could I have gotten mercury toxicity? There have been two reported cases of mercury poisonings in pregnant females, here in Asheville, N.C., from tuna and swordfish. Remember those vaccines you had when you were younger? They were preserved with mercury; as are flu shots now.

Commercial Chelation

Intravenous chelation is controversial, as is oral chelation, except in the true case of extremely high blood levels of heavy metals; in which case the metal usually nearly kills the patient before we find the toxic metal.

Chelation From Our Diet

Our current environment, food and water supplies expose us to heavy metal toxins that can influence our brains over time. There are natural "chelators" in nature. Chelating (pronounced key-layting) agents (both natural and synthetic) are substances which can chemically bond with or chelate (from the Greek chele claw) metals, minerals or chemical toxins from the body. The chelating agent actually encircles a mineral or metal ion and carries it from the body via the urine or feces. Chelation is especially helpful in eliminating toxic metals mercury, lead, cadmium, nickel, arsenic, aluminum, etc.

Nature To The Rescue

Vitamin C is a natural chelator. Vitamin C (Ascorbic Acid) is one of the most important antioxidants; it can easily enter the blood brain barrier and reach the brain cells, where it is needed most. This means that you can increase the level of vitamin C in your brain by eating more fresh fruits and veggies. It is also a very effective detoxifier of heavy metals and chemical poisons. Vitamin C has detoxifying actions on lead, mercury, carbon monoxide, sulfur dioxide, various carcinogens, bacterial toxins and poisons; and it protects us from benzene exposure.

Cilantro

Cilantro (Chinese Parsley) - has been shown in clinical trials and research to mobilize and effectively remove mercury, tin, lead, aluminum and other toxic metals stored in the brain and spinal cord. This is a revolutionary discovery and makes Cilantro the first known substance that mobilizes mercury from the CNS (Central Nervous System).

Cilantro Pesto

1 clove of garlic1/2 cup of almonds, cashews, or other nuts
1 cup packed fresh cilantro leaves
2 tablespoons lemon juice
6 tablespoons olive oil

Put the cilantro and olive oil in blender and process until the cilantro is chopped. Add the rest of the ingredients and process to a lumpy paste. (You may need to add a touch of hot water and scrape the sides of the blender). You can change the consistency by altering the amount of olive oil and lemon juice, but keep the 3:1 ratio of oil to juice. (It freezes well, so you can make several batches at once.)

Amino Acids Help Too!

L-Glutathione can cross the blood-brain barrier and remove mercury, cadmium and other toxic metals from the brain. It is a powerful free radical scavenger and antioxidant that removes unwanted substances from the body. It is found in protein rich plant foods like soy, nuts, wheat, brown rice and beans.

L-Cysteine acts as a reducing agent that prevents the oxidation of sensitive tissues that leads to aging and cancer. It also helps protect against the effects of alcohol consumption, protects cell membranes against lipid peroxidation, and detoxifies pesticides, plastics, hydrocarbons, and other chemicals. This sulfurous amino acid is critical for the detoxification of heavy metals and xenobiotics (estrogen-like, non-polar, fat-soluble chemical substances that may interfere with normal estrogen functions and play a role in creating cancer). L-Cysteine helps protect the liver and brain from damage due to alcohol, drugs, and toxic compounds in cigarette smoke. L-cysteine chelates mercury and arsenic, and its antioxidant effects are appropriate for countering all metals. It is a potent sulfhydryl antioxidant, heavy metal scavenger, and liver protector. The body can synthesize cysteine from the aminoacid methionine but it is also found in high protein foods such as wheat, broccoli, garlic, onions and red peppers.

L-Lysine also detoxifies heavy metals. L-lysine is lipotropic, meaning that it has a high affinity for fats (lipids) and assists in fat metabolism. It is involved in the structural repair of damaged collagen in arteriosclerotic blood vessels. L-lysine is used as an aid to improve athletic performance and is required for collagen synthesis. Good sources of lysine are lima beans, potatoes, soy milk and brewer's yeast.

L-Methionine is an essential amino acid that helps remove heavy metals from the body and protects against the toxic effects of radiation. This sulfur-containing amino acid is critical for the detoxification of heavy metals and xenobiotics. It assists in the breakdown of fat, and helps prevent fatty build-up in the liver and arteries that might obstruct blood flow to the brain, heart, and kidneys. It is a powerful antioxidant that is also beneficial to people with chemical allergies. L-Methionine chelates lead, and is effective in preventing liver damage and supporting liver functioning. Methionine is found in good quantities in beans, garlic, lentils, onions, yogurt and seeds.

Chlorella

Chlorella is seaweed, or a type of algae that grows in water. Chlorella is known to promote the elimination of heavy metals from the body, as does barley green and wheat grass. The chlorella algae cell wall absorbs rather large amounts of toxic metals. Either the specific combination of amino acids, the chlorella derived growth factor, or some other unknown mechanism leads to the mobilization of mercury and other toxins from within the cell. It appears to mobilize mercury deposits within the brain. Chlorella is a nutritious source of chlorophyll that has also been found to cleanse the bloodstream and be a protective agent against the effects of ultraviolet radiation.

Other Natural Chelators

Garlic chelates cadmium, lead and mercury within the body. Spirulina-based products help chelate, too. The herb, yellow dock root, is a specific chelator for aluminum. Selenium chelates heavy metals such as cadmium, lead, mercury and silver.

Stiff Vessels From Deficiencies

The male's prostate gland requires high levels of zinc and contains some of the body's highest stores of this mineral. Cadmium, a known carcinogen, seems to concentrate in prostate, breast and uterus tissue, and seems to mimics estrogen.

Your body's cells are constantly being repaired or replaced. Your body uses what raw materials are available at the time of the cell's repair or building new cells. Your cells in your arteries require zinc to help flexibility and cell wall strength. But, if zinc is deficient in the diet, the toxic metal cadmium could be used instead, if it's available. The chemical structure of zinc and cadmium are similar enough for the body to do the substitution and continue functioning, though at a less efficient level. The loss of flexibility in your blood vessels may cause high blood pressure and ultimately a stroke, and the fragile vessel is more susceptible to damage, leading to blockages and cardiovascular disease.

Eat Right!

Be sure that you get a steady and constant supply of trace minerals and nutrients. You are what you eat. Avoid environmental exposure to toxic metals. Your body can replace most toxic building blocks as it repairs and rebuilds, if you supply it with the right materials.

Known Mineral Antagonists

MINERAL	TOXIC METAL
Calcium	Lead
Zinc	Cadmium
Sulfur/Molybdenum	Copper
Selenium	Mercury, lead, silver and cadmium

Think Right!

As we do all we can to rid ourselves of potentially harmful toxic heavy metals, we should do all we can in our lives for Christ's sake; as in the early Advent revival. "The assurance of the Savior's approval was more necessary to them than their daily food; and if a cloud darkened their minds, they did not rest until it was swept away." Great Controversy, 1911:403

References:
Marcus, S. Lead Toxicity. eMedicine. October 4, 2004. http://www. emedicine.com/emerg/topic293.htm .
Williams, D., *"Brain Drain,"* Alternatives, August 2005, Vol.11, No.2:10-14.
Achanzar W, Diwan B, Liu J, et al., Cadmium-induced Malignant Transformation of Human Prostate Epithelial Cells, Cancer Res 2001;61(2):455-458.
Brys M, Nawrocka A, Miekos E, et al., Zinc and Cadmium Analysis in Human Prostate neoplasms. Biol Trace Elem Res., 1997;59(1-3):145-152.
Omura, Y., Cilantro and Mercury Removal, Acupunct Electrother Res.,1996;21 (2):133-60 and Acupnct Electrother Res.,1995;20 (3-4):195-229.

HEADACHES - MIGRAINES

Approximately 60 million Americans suffer from chronic headaches, and 28 million of them suffer from migraines.

Headache Vs. Migraine

Ordinary (tension) headaches are usually caused by muscle tension at the back of your head and neck. Migraines differ from ordinary headaches because they are caused by changes in the size of the blood vessels supplying your brain. While the exact cause of each kind of headache remains in debate, most researchers believe that a migraine attack involves the constriction of the arteries in your brain, followed by their reactive widening (dilation) pressing against your non-expandable skull. A migraine headache is a throbbing or pulsating headache that is often on one or both sides of the head associated with or without an aura, nausea, vomiting, sensitivity to light (photophobia), sound, smells, sleep disturbance, unusual tiredness, mood changes and depression. They may occur at any age, but usually begin between the ages of 10 and 40and diminish after age 50. Some people experience several migraines a month, while others have only a few migraines throughout their lifetime. Approximately 75% of migraine sufferers are women.

Four Phases Of Migraines

1) **Prodrome.** The "prodrome" phase warns that a migraine is coming. Symptoms include changes in your mental state, such as irritability or confusion, and physical signs such as thirst or diarrhea. One out of every four migraine sufferers experiences prodrome symptoms as early as 24 hours before the migraine pain attacks.
2) **Aura.** A neurological warning (aura) can be experienced 10 to 60 minutes before a headache. Most auras are visual, like bright shimmering

lights around objects or at the edges of the field of vision (called scintillating scotomas) or zigzag lines, castles (teichopsia), wavy images, or hallucinations. Some experience temporary vision loss. Non-visual auras include motor weakness, speech or language abnormalities, dizziness, vertigo, tingling or numbness (parasthesia) of the face, tongue, or extremities-just like a stroke. About one in five migraine sufferers experience auras.

3) **Pain**. The pain phase can last from several hours to 72 hours.

4) **Resolution.** After a migraine, many people experience deep fatigue and general malaise for up to 24 hours.

Rebound Headaches

Rebound migraines stem from too much caffeine, prescription migraine drugs or non-prescription pain relievers. Taking something almost daily, or as little as three days a week can cause a sufferer to get in a cycle called "rebound." Your body becomes accustomed to the headache treatment and without it you go through withdrawal, your headache returns, and you take more meds. Use the '2-5 Rebound Rule:' treat your migraine for 2 days and then don't take anything for at least 5 days thereafter.

Menstrual/Hormonal Migraines

Menstrual migraines can occur just prior to or during menstruation. These headaches are related to hormonal changes and often do not occur, or lessen during pregnancy. Some women develop migraines for the first time during pregnancy or after menopause. Birth control pills as well as hormone replacement therapy peri-menopausal or during menopause can trigger migraines in some women.

Ocular Migraines

Eye migraines occur when blood flow to the brain responsible for vision (visual cortex or occipital lobe) is disturbed, resulting in ophthalmic or ocular migraines that produce visual symptoms, even without a headache. They have nothing to do with your eye. Characteristically you will see a small, enlarging blind spot (scotoma) in your central vision with bright, flickering lights (scintillations) or a shimmering zigzag line (metamorphopsia) inside the blind spot. The blind spot usually enlarges and may move across your field of vision. The entire migraine visual episode can last between 2 and 30 minutes.

Silent Migraines

A silent migraine has many features of a regular migraine (may have an aura), but is without the actual headache pain. It is frequently mistaken for other illnesses, because a person may experience visual, auditory and speech problems.

Cluster Migraines

Cluster headaches are a rare type of headache, affecting 0.1% of the population. An estimated 85% of cluster headache sufferers are men. The average age of cluster headache sufferers is 28-30 years of age, although these headaches may begin in childhood. Half of these sufferers' headaches can be triggered by alcohol. Treatment usually includes anti-inflammatories, i.e., prednisone.

Sinus Headaches

A sinus headache can occur when the sinuses become plugged or congested. The sinuses are the bony, air-filled cavities in the face/head that connect to the nose through small openings. During a cold or allergy attack, the openings can become blocked by excess mucus and may become infected. People who have an injury to the bones in the nose, a deformity of the nose, or any condition that hinders the draining of the sinuses, may be at greater risk of getting a sinus headache. Increasing your water intake to one ounce per kilogram (2.2 pounds) of your bodyweight daily will help thin the nasal mucous in your nose and diminish your sinus headache.

Tension Headaches

Tension headaches are the most common type of headache and are usually caused by muscle tightness at the back of your head and neck. As many as 90% of adults have had or will have tension headaches.

Triggers For Migraines

Emotional stress, changes in normal sleep pattern, extreme fatigue, specific foods and beverages, caffeine intake or withdrawal, skipping meals- fasting, changing weather conditions, exercise, smoking, bright and flickering lights, and odors can all trigger migraines. Natural chemicals in foods, food additives, artificial sweeteners and beverages, food additives/preservatives like nitrates and nitrites found in ham, sausage and other processed or cured meats, salads in salad bars, monosodium glutamate (MSG) in Chinese food and alcohol, specifically the impurities in alcohol or byproducts your body produces as it metabolizes alcohol, can all act as triggers for your migraine.

Tyramine Induced Migraines

Foods containing tyramine, a vaso-active amino acid, can cause migraines. Tyramine is an intermediate product in the conversion of tyrosine (an amino acid present in many proteins) to epinephrine (an active hormone produced by the inner portion of the adrenal gland).

Specific tyramine/food triggers include: **Aged cheeses**: blue cheese, mozzarella, feta, cheddar, Parmesan; **Alcohol:** red wine, beer, whiskey, champagne; **Caffeine:** coffee, chocolate, tea, colas, sodas; **Processed meats:** pepperoni, salami, liverwurst, bacon, hot dogs, luncheon meats, mincemeat pie; **Bread** and other baked goods; **Dried fruits**-like raisins; smoked or dried fish, potato chips, pizza, peanuts, chicken livers, onions, olives, Fava or broad beans, sauerkraut, pickles, any fermented soy products (ie miso, soy sauce, teriyaki sauce), any kind of nut, avocados, and canned soups.

Avoid Your Migraine Triggers

- Watch what you eat and drink.
- If you get a headache, write down any food or drink you had before getting it. If you see a pattern over time, eliminate that item!
- Eat regularly. Skipping meals can trigger migraines in some people.
- Cut out caffeine. Excess caffeine (in any food or drink) can cause migraines.
- Avoid artificial sweeteners.
- Get regular sleep. Changes in your normal sleep habits can cause migraines. Being overly tired can also trigger migraines.
- Learn to cope with stress. Emotional upsets and stressful events are common migraine triggers. Anxiety, worry, fatigue, and excitement can intensify a migraine's severity. Learn to cope with stress better -through prayer, counseling, and relaxation.

OTC (Over The Counter) Treatments For Headaches

Butterbur (Petasites hybridus) is an extremely popular herbal remedy in Germany, where it is widely used as a preventative for migraines. It also works for allergies. Butterbur inhibits toxic chemicals called leukotrienes, which are released during the inflammatory process. It has also been found to help regulate the degree of widening of the arteries in the brain (Forsch Kompl Klass 2003, 10(1):41-44). The recommended dosage is one 50mg standardized butterbur extract capsule taken twice a day with meals.

Peppermint oil/Capsicum oil. First make sure you are hydrated and avoid caffeine. Water is the best for headaches. Place 4 drops of Peppermint oil on a cotton ball and rub the oil into your temples and the back of your neck. Next, place 4 drops of Capsicum oil on a new cotton ball and rub this oil in the same places that you did with the Peppermint. Using an electronic massager or a friend, massage your temples and the back of your neck with enough force to feel the effects but not enough to cause more pain. Use your middle finger and index finger to massage in circular motions on your temples. Continue drinking water and rest your eyes if necessary. Your head should feel better almost instantly.

Capsaicin, the natural chemical extracted from hot pepper plants (the active ingredient in pepper spray), opens up the sinus passages and blunts pain pathways. It can be used both topically and orally for sinus headaches, cluster headaches and migraines.

Co-enzyme Q-10 is an essential element of the mitochondrial electron transport chain and cellular respiration. It is found in soybeans, olive, grapeseeds, sunflower, rice bran, coconut, peanuts, walnuts, sesame seeds, pistachio nuts, hazelnuts, almond, parsley, broccoli, cauliflower, spinach, Chinese cabbage, avocado, blackcurrant, and strawberries. Coenzyme Q-10 can be blocked by cholesterol lowering statins. A 50% decrease in headaches was seen after 12 weeks of taking 150-600 mg of Co Enzyme Q-10 daily. (Rozen, TD, Oshinsky, ML, Gebeline, CA, Bradley, KC, Young, WB, Shechter, AL & Silberstein, SD. "Open label trial of coenzyme Q-10 as a migraine preventive." Cephalalgia 22 (2)137-141.)

Feverfew (Tanacetym parthenium). Researchers working at the Department of Neurology, University of Essen, in Germany, studied the effects of feverfew on a group of 147 migraine sufferers. At the end of the four-week study, the researchers found that the patients taking feverfew experienced a significant reduction in the frequency and severity of their migraines compared to those in the placebo group. Not only that, but pain, nausea, vomiting and sensitivity to light were also significantly reduced following treatment with feverfew (Cephalalgia 2002, 22(7):523-532). Another study found that feverfew can reduce migraine frequency in up to two thirds of cases (Brit. Med. J. 291:569-73, 1985). The recommended dosage is one 125 mg feverfew capsule taken once a day.

Caffeine can be both beneficial and harmful for a headache sufferer. It can serve as a treatment or be addictive causing insomnia, irritability, anxiety, palpitations and headaches. Caffeine can cause withdrawal or rebound headaches. Cut it out.

Avoid Sugar. Many migraine sufferers report experiencing an attack shortly after eating too much sugary food (Headache Quart 1997,8(4):319-329). In addition to sweets and sugar, refined carbohydrates also cause your blood sugar levels to quickly rise. This interferes with the normal actions of various neurotransmitters, such as serotonin, which are implicated in causing migraines.

Powdered Ginger 400-600 mg, 1/3 teaspoon, every four hours (total 4000 mg-6000 mg a day), fresh, tea, or capsule, improves headaches by decreasing nausea, platelet adhesion and inflammatory prostaglandins.

Magnesium. Migraines have been linked to the deficiency of the trace mineral magnesium. Magnesium helps the transmission of chemical messages from the brain to the arteries and helps control the degree of arterial dilatation (widening). Several hospitals in Canada and Germany use magnesium supplements as a standard treatment for acute migraines and prevention. The dose is 200 mg of magnesium citrate capsules taken twice a day. Avoid if you have renal failure or diarrhea.

Omega-3. In one small study at the University of Cincinnati, high dose Omega-3 reduced migraines by 40-50%. Walnuts (Black and English), pecans, raw seeds, freshly ground flaxseed, and fish oil are sources of Omega-3.

Melatonin is a hormone produced in the brain's pineal gland; it helps regulate sleep-wake cycles. Imbalances in the level of melatonin in the body may be related to headaches like migraines and cluster headaches. A Brazilian study found a 75% decrease in headaches if the individual took 3 mg of melatonin before bedtime each day.

B Vitamins are good for preventing migraines. Vitamins B2, B3 and B6 help prevent vasoconstriction (narrowing of the arteries) and also inhibit blood platelet clumping (micro clots/scabs) which can occur during a migraine attack (Cephalalgia 1994, 14(5):328-329). Vitamin B12 increases synaptic function of your nerves, which decreases the inappropriate brain blood vessel response in a migraine.

Prescription Treatments For Migraines

Triptans/Ergotamine

Triptans* and ergotamine** products constrict the blood vessels in your brain, reducing your migraine or cluster headache. These work by stimulating serotonin (selective serotonin receptor agonist).

**Imitrex (sumatriptan), almotriptan (Axert), eletriptan (Relpax), frovatriptan (Frova), rizatriptan (Maxalt), naratriptan (Amerge), zolmitriptan (Zomig),*

*** ergotamine: methysergide (Sansert), ergotamine (Ergomar, Ergostat, Cafergot, Ercaf, Wigraine), dihydroergotamine (D.H.E. 45, Migranal NasalSpray), ergonovine (Ergotrate), or methylergonovine (Methergine).*

Beta and Calcium Channel Blockers

Beta (1 and 2 receptor) blockers (Inderal-popranolol) are usually used for hypertension, angina pectoris and cardiac arrhythmia, but taken daily can block and dampen the effect of migraine triggers. Calcium Channel blockers (like verapamil) are believed to benefit migraine suffers from their anti vaso-constrictor activity, inhibition of platelet aggregation, serotonin release, and/or serotonin and histamine receptor blockade.

Anticonvulsants (Seizure Medicine)

Seizure medications are used to control epilepsy, but these meds are also used to prevent migraine headaches. These include: Phenytoin (Dilantin), Carbamazepine (Tegretol), Divalproex sodium (Depakote), Gabapentin (Neurotin), and Topiramate (Topamax).

Botox

Since 1992, Botox, the same bacteria that causes deadly food poisoning, has been used in purified and diluted form to temporarily paralyze the muscles that bring the eye brows together, thereby eliminating wrinkles in this region. Doctors injecting botulinum toxin A in the upper third of the face for treatment of cosmetic frown lines had their patients, who coincidentally suffered from migraines, report headache relief.

Cervical/Cranial Surgery

A surprisingly large number of my patients that have had cervical spine surgery for disc disease/stenosis or foramen ovale (the big opening in the bottom of your skull)- Chiari Malformation surgery have found relief from their lifetime of headaches.

The Headache Not To Ignore!

Severe headache, or medical emergency? Know your personal headache symptoms. Rarely are headaches as serious as a tumor, stroke, encephalitis, meningitis or aneurysm (blood vessel rupture).

Symptoms to watch for: paralysis of the arms or legs, tingling, numbness, confusion, dizziness, double vision, slurred speech, trouble finding words, weakness, especially on one side of the face/body or the worst headache you ever had.

Prayer

We have neighbors that regularly kneel down together and pray when they develop a migraine headache. Humbling oneself before our merciful God does wonders for their headaches. You need to try it.

References:

MIGRAINE- Google Health, Mayo Clinic.com, Medline Plus, WebMD, Wikipedia, Web 05-07 to 12-10.

HELICOBACTER PYLORI

- Do You Have a Non-Healing Peptic Ulcer?
- The Truth About Mastic Gum Resin

I was approached in the hall this week by one of the hospital's employees asking about her father. He had just been diagnosed with H. Pylori (Helicobacter Pylori) of the stomach and refused to have another round of antibiotics. "Is there anything that he can use that is not prescription?" I was asked. "Yes, there is a very successful over-the-counter treatment of H Pylori without the danger of using recurrent rounds of antibiotics to eradicate this bug."

How Can H. Pylori Affect Me?

H. Pylori are gram-negative rods that can cause open sores (ulcers) in your stomach and small intestine. H. pylori infection can irritate the lining of the stomach, causing inflammation (gastritis). H. pylori infection is a strong risk factor for certain types of stomach cancer, including adenocarcinoma and gastric mucosa-associated lymphoid tissue (MALT) lymphoma. More than 50% of the world's population have a H. pylori infection, but over 80% of individuals infected with the bacterium are asymptomatic. Yet in others, H. pylori can lead to serious complications. Signs or symptoms that can occur with H. pylori infection (as well as other causes) include: an ache or burning pain in your abdomen, frequent burping, bloating, weight loss, severe or persistent abdominal pain, difficulty swallowing, bloody or black tarry stools, bloody or black vomit or vomit that looks like coffee grounds.

How Does H. Pylori Survive The Stomach Acid?

To colonize the stomach, H. pylori must survive the acidic pH and burrow into the mucus of the stomach's epithelial cell layer. The bacterium has flagella (mobile tails) and moves through the stomach and drills into the mucoid lining of the stomach or bowel. H. pylori senses the pH gradient within the mucus layer by chemo taxis and swims away from the acidic contents towards the more neutral pH environment of the epithelial cell surface. H. pylori induces inflammation and locally high levels of TNF α and interleukin 6. That's why high doses of omega-3 (flax seed oil, walnuts, fish oil, etc) helps GI symptoms because it down regulates levels of TNF α and interleukin 6.

How Can I Get H. Pylori?

H. pylori is passed from person to person through direct contact with saliva or fecal matter. H. pylori can also be spread through untreated water and house flies. You may have the infection for years before you have any symptoms. I believe some people are genetically more likely to get a H pylori infection than others. What's the most common cause of recurrent symptoms after successful treatment? Getting exposed to the bacterium again!

How Do I Find Out If I Have A H. Pylori Infection?

1) The most common way is by pricking your finger for a blood test. The test strips turn positive or negative in 15 minutes, just like a pregnancy test. **2**) During a breath test, you drink a solution that contains radioactive carbon molecules. If you have an H. pylori infection, the radioactive carbon is released when the solution is broken down in your stomach. Your body absorbs the radioactive carbon and expels it when you exhale. You exhale into a bag and your doctor uses a special device to detect the radioactive carbon. **3**) A laboratory test called a stool antigen test looks for foreign proteins (antigens) associated with H. pylori infection in your stool. **4**) During an endoscopy exam, your doctor threads a long flexible tube equipped with a tiny camera (endoscope) down your throat and esophagus and into your stomach and duodenum. Using this instrument, your doctor can view any irregularities in your upper digestive tract and remove tissue samples (biopsy). These samples are analyzed for H. pylori infection.

Doctors Demonized For The Right Diagnosis

H. pylori was first discovered in the stomachs of patients with gastritis & stomach ulcers by Dr. Barry J. Marshall and Dr. J. Robin Warren of Perth, Western Australia, but veterinarians long knew that a round of antibiotics would cure a animal that was not eating (1920). Medical thinking felt that the stomach acid (equal to car-battery acid) would kill any bacteria in it. When I was in Medical School (1977-1980) the standard treatment for recurrent ulcers was a gastric resection and vagotomy. This removed 3/4 of one's stomach and cut the nerves to their stomach. Drs. Marshall & Warren "re-wrote" the text-books for what caused gastritis & gastric ulcers and received so much vitriol (bitterly abusive outcry) from doctors and scientists around the world that it is reported they had to go into hiding. They finally received their reward: the 2005 Nobel Prize for Medicine & Physiology.

How To Treat H. Pylori

An increasing number of infected individuals are found to have antibiotic-resistant bacteria. This results in initial treatment failure (clarithromycin and amoxicillin for 14 days) and requires additional rounds of antibiotic therapy or quadruple therapy, which adds Bismuth subsalicylate (Pepto-Bismol four times a day for 14 days-makes your stool black) and proton pump inhibitors-PPI (suppress acids by shutting down "pumps" in acid producing cells-twice a day for 14 days):omeprazole (Prilosec), lansoprazole (Prevacid), pantoprazole (Protonix), rabeprazole (Aciphex) and esomeprazole (Nexium). For the treatment of clarithromycin (Biaxin) resistant strains of H. pylori doctors uselevofloxacin (Levaquin) as part of the therapy. Variations of the therapy include using a different proton pump inhibitor, adding Pepto-Bismol (the bismuth suppresses the H. pylori) or replacing amoxicillin with metronidazole (Flagyl) for people who are allergic to penicillin.

So What Do I Recommend?

I recommend first a two week round of antibiotics, with a PPI twice a day for 14 days and Pepto-Bismol 4 times a day (one tbsp or tablet = one dose) for two weeks. If you do not respond, don't want antibiotics or the symptoms reoccur, I would substitute the antibiotic portion of the protocol with Mastica capsules two 250 mg twice a day (total at least one gram daily), on an empty stomach, for 14 days and include the other two treatments (PPI and Bismuth). Mastica (mastic gum resin) can be found at any health food store. Mastica works very well and resolves many of my patient's chest pains (after we have proven the chest pain is noncardiac). I have some patients that will use this treatment several times a year for relief of their recurring symptoms.

Mastic Gum Resin

Mastica is the resin obtained from the Pistacia lentiscus tree (an evergreen shrub from the pistachio tree family) which is grown on the island of Chios in Greece. It has been used for a variety of gastric ailments in Mediterranean and Mideast countries for at least 3,000 years. Traditionally used as a health food in Greece, a 1998 study reported in the New England Journal of Medicine supports mastica's part in eliminating H. pylori. Isn't God wonderful for creating from nature a treatment for man's upset stomachs!

References:

Graham DY, et al. Helicobacter pylori. In: Feldman M, et al. Sleisenger & Fordtran's Gastrointestinal and Liver Disease: Pathophysiology, Diagnosis, Management. 8th ed. Philadelphia, Pa.: Saunders Elsevier; 2006. http://www.mdconsult.com/das/book/body/134273666-3/0/1389/0.html. Accessed April 28, 2009.

Fuccio L, et al. Treatment of Helicobacter pylori infection. BMJ. 2008;337:746.

H. pylori and peptic ulcer. National Institute for Diabetes and Digestive and Kidney Diseases. http://digestive.niddk.nih.gov/ddiseases/pubs/hpylori/index.htm. Accessed April 29, 2009.

Talley NJ, et al. Gastric cancer consensus conference recommends Helicobacter pylori screening and treatment in asymptomatic personsfrom high-risk populations to prevent gastric cancer. American Journal of Gastroenterology. 2008;103:510.

1998-2010 Mayo Foundation for Medical Education and Research (MFMER). Mastic Gum kills H. Pylori, NEJM 1998 Dec 24;339(26):1946.

HOPE AND YOUR HEALTH

-Can A Positive Attitude Be Learned? -Are You Always Grumpy? -Are You A Pessimist Or An optimist? -

Happiness Is An Inside Job!

"A merry heart doeth good like a medicine: but a broken spirit drieth the bones." Proverbs 17:22

"Rejoice in the Lord always; again I say, Rejoice." Philippians 4:4

Happiness Is A State Of Mind

Why would God tell us to be happy, if we couldn't direct our minds to be cheerful? Researchers for years have thought that hope and optimism are keys to a longer life. Multiple prospective cohort studies have suggested that feeling hopeful is a predictor of well-being and physical health. Dispositional optimism, positive expectancies for one's future or better classified as 'hope,' has been studied in association with cardiovascular death in the healthy elderly. There was a 50% lower risk of cardiovascular death in the optimistic elderly over 15 year period, than in the hopeless or depressive personality type. Interestingly, receiving either good or bad news didn't change the outlook in the optimistic group. This supports the idea that dispositional optimism is a relatively constant trait of an individual's personality and is sufficiently stable over long periods of time, thus lowering the hyper-adrenaline death risk over time.

D Type Personality Predicts Death After Stent Implantation

People that are distressed or have negative outlook on life (Type D personality, as opposed to an A type personality) have been shown to independently predict adverse outcomes when they have ischemic heart disease. The prognostic power of the Type D personality equals that of having a poorly functioning heart pump, even if they have a normal appearing heart. Incidentally, the stent type did not make a difference. Poorer prognosis was seen in as little as 9 months. Type D personalities had higher circulating cytokines (inflammatory markers) and more abnormal levels of epinephrine and nor epinephrine than those that were happy with life. Positive mental health can make the difference between life and death.

Symptoms Of Norepinephrine Abnormality

Symptoms of norepinephrine imbalance include aggression, anger, tension, irritability, rage, cravings, increased appetite and manic like symptoms.

Mind Over Matter

You've heard it said, "Mind over matter." How can you normalize your cytokine and adrenalin levels?

1. Laughter normalizes cytokine and adrenalin levels.
2. Exercise normalizes cytokine and adrenalin levels.
3. Increase your fiber intake, natural foods and raw food choices. During stress or duress avoid processed food and sugar. Emotional illness may be rooted in a poor diet and nutrition.
4. Take a walk outside. Stop and take a deep breath. Close your eyes and remember the sights, smells and sounds around you. Recall these memories throughout a tough day.
5. Prayerful meditation normalizes cytokine and adrenalin levels. "Pray without ceasing."

So How Do You Become Optimistic?

Can 'hope' be learned or taught? After my near-death experience, everything was placed in perspective. Live each day to its fullest, as if it were your last. With my Crohn's Disease, there are days that I have no energy, and others when I feel better, and then I do too much. Here's what I do: find pleasure in the little things of life; enjoy the sounds (birds, music), colors (the flowers, the different shades of green in the grass and trees), the textures of life in general. The happiest people are those who are able to avoid constant arguments, let go of resentments, and therefore build close relationships with God and man. We are told to teach children to be industrious, love God supremely, and remember the little courtesies of life; these things are essential to happiness.[1] If we can teach children these things, then we can re-direct our minds to do the same.

What *Won't* Make You Happy

Remember, being unhappy can be a habit, just as easily as learning to be happy.

What doesn't make you happy is:

1. Money.[2] Ask a big lottery winner.

2. Intelligence[3] Look up the life of King Solomon.
3. Amusement.[4]
4. Anything that gratifies self.[5]

What *Will* Make You Happy

What are some sources of happiness that will change our outlook on life?

1. Focus on the positive. *"All things work together for good to those that love Him."* Romans.8:28
2. Fix your mind on cheerful things.[6] Smile; if you have to, fake it. A smile will lift your mood.
3. Be agreeable.
4. Focus on the now. Have single-mindedness.
5. Helping others and making other happy[7] [8]
6. Stave off loneliness.
7. Feed your sense of hope. We sing of having this hope; hope in the future; that believing something better is in store for us.

What To Do With Worry

"Worry is blind, and cannot discern the future; but Jesus sees the end from the beginning. In every difficulty He has His way prepared to bring relief. Our heavenly Father has thousand ways to provide for us, of which we know nothing. Those who accept the one principle of making the service and honor of God supreme will find perplexes vanish, and a plain path before their feet."[9]

References:

Giltay, E.J., *"Dispositional Optimism And the Risk Of Cardiovascular Death,"* The Zutphen Elderly Study; Arch Intern Med, Vol.166, Feb 27, 2006:431-436.

Pederen, S.S., *"Type D Personality Predicts Death Or Myocardial Infraction After Bare Metal Stent Or Sirolimus-Eluting Stent Implantation,"* J Am Coll Cardiol, 2004;44:997-1001.

Tan, S., *"Laughter Is Good For You,"* Loma Linda University, Bottom Line, 11/15/2000:9.

Cheraskin,E., *"Emotional Illness May Be Rooted In Poor Diet And Nutrition,"* Nutrition Health Review, Spring 2002:7.

1 White, E., "Aim at High Points in Character Development," Child Guidance:189
2 White, E., "Laboring For Special Classes," Evangelism:556
3 White, E., Testimonies To The Church;Vol.2:305
4 White, E., Testimonies To Ministers And Gospel Workers:103
5 White, E., Child Guidance:206
6 White, E., Ministry Of Healing:248
7 White, E., "The Acts Of The Apostles:12
8 White, E., Testimonies To The Church;Vol.2:248 9White, E., Desire Of Ages:330

ARE PLASTICS MAKING YOU SICK?

- Tiny Bits, Big Problems
- Is It Safe To Heat Food In Plastic?

Are You Exposed To Synthetic Estrogens?

Plastics are one of the greatest inventions of all time. Modern life depends on them. They are in everything from appliances, insulation, cars, clothing, to food and water containers, etc. Are plastics making us sick? Which ones, if any?

Going Green

So you're trying to be green and reuse your plastic water and juice bottles, butter/margarine tubs and plastic food storage containers. STOP IT!! 85% of the rest of the world throws away this stuff without recycling.* Recycle it, don't re-use it.

BPA = A Hormone Disrupter

Bisphenol-A (BPA) is an endocrine/estrogen-like disrupting chemical in animal studies. At low doses, BPA causes cell and tissue changes that can cause early puberty, behavior problems, breast and prostate cancer, altered immune function and metabolic problems. The CDC reported in 2008 that 93% of tested individuals had BPA in their urine. Higher levels were seen in woman and children. It was first synthesized in 1891; BPA came into use as a synthetic estrogen in 1936. It was passed over for a stronger synthetic estrogen diethylstilbestrol (DES) in the 1940s.** In the 1950s, chemists discovered that, combined with phosgene (used during World War I as a toxic gas) and other compounds, BPA yielded the hard, clear, lightweight, polycarbonate plastic of shatter-resistant headlights, eyeglass lenses, DVDs and baby bottles. In the US, BPA has been in the lining of food and beverage cans since 1963. Japan has replaced BPA to line their cans since 1997 with natural resin. BPA is crucial in making polyester. In the U.S. alone more than 2.3 billion pounds (1.04 million metric tons) of BPA is manufactured annually.

How Do You Get BPA In Your Body?

BPA is found in those indestructible water bottles (not the disposable ones), sippy cups, pacifiers, beauty supplies, toys, running shoes, etc. During the manufacturing process, not all BPA gets locked into chemical bonds. That residual BPA can work itself free, especially when the plastic is heated, whether it's a Nalgene bottle in the dishwasher or hot car or a food container in the microwave. BPA can also be picked up by humans in the soil, water and dust. Putting boiling water in new and old BPA-type polycarbonate bottles released 55 times more BPA. Acidic foods, like tomatoes, and fatty foods (like gravy) cause more leaching of BPA from their cans. The Environment Working Group found BPA in more than half of the 97 food cans it tested, with the highest levels coming from chicken soup, infant formula and ravioli. The FDA estimates that the average adult American consumes, on average, a cumulative 11 micrograms of BPA a day through diet, mostly from canned foods. Is that too much? Most adults process it in less than a day; it is broken down into glucuronide. But babies and fetuses do not excrete it quickly.

Human Studies

Studies in humans are limited, but the American Medical Association (JAMA) found high levels of BPA was associated with heart disease, diabetes Type 2, and abnormal liver enzymes. This did not prove that BPA caused these problems. Most manufacturer and retailers are phasing out BPA and phthalates in their products, including Wal-Mart, CVS, Nike and Proctor and Gamble. Canada has called it a "toxic substance." California and other states are trying to ban polycarbonate with BPA.

What Makes The Poison?

Toxicologists function under the well known theory that "the dose makes the poison"– the more chemical you ingest, the sicker you get. That's why the FDA states that you are safe. You would have to ingest 500 pounds of canned foods and beverages a day to reach the safety standards set for BPA in the US and Europe. But if you are not directly poisoned, could you be harmed by BPA and phthalates? BPA and phthalates are endocrine disruptors–chemicals that interfere with, mimic, shut down or modify the chemical signals that regulate everything from metabolism and reproduction to our bodies' response to stress. Therefore, by theory, tiny doses can cause problems if the exposure is at a critical time in development. SO, the volume of the foreign chemical may not be as important as "the timing makes the poison." Not until recently could these tiny doses even be measured. Is it possible that early exposure to chemicals like BPA makes us grow up to be chubby, infertile and prone to sickness as children and adults? This is the thinking of many in the medical community who feel vaccines, given at the wrong time, may trigger autism.

Phthalates

BPA contains phthalates (a wide range of chemicals). Phthalates are in car dashboards, vinyl shower curtains, raincoats, and even your rubber ducky, to make them pliable. Phthalates are in beauty products, like nail polish, to prevent chipping. 75% of 2450 men, women and children tested (ages 6 to 85) had seven different phthalates in their urine. Children had the highest chemical levels. Lower sperm counts and other reproductive abnormalities were found in men with the highest levels of certain phthalates in their urine. In girls, phthalate levels seven times higher than the control group correlated with early puberty (breasts at age 2 to 6) in Puerto Rico. Early puberty has been linked to cancer (breast and prostate). People with higher than average phthalate levels tended to have larger waists and increased insulin resistance. Scientists suggest that higher levels of BPA and phthalates during fetal and childhood development could affect the brain structure, function and behavior, like causing attention deficient hyperactivity disorder (ADHD). It does in rats and mice. High BPA levels can interfere with chemotherapy.

Xeno Estrogens

Further complicating this issue is the stew of other estrogen-mimicking chemicals to which we are routinely exposed. Synthetic xeno estrogens (one of many hormone disrupters) not only comes from BPA and phthalates, but are released from other plastic products like dental sealants; they are in makeup, hair spray, shampoo, pesticides and meats, to name a few. Europe has outlawed hormone treated meat, including estradiol (one form of estrogen***), but it is routinely used in cows in North America, Australia, New Zealand and Argentina. North America has the highest rate of breast and prostate cancer in the world. How much estrogen from meat are Americans getting? The FDA says very little; the European researchers say a lot. Investigators today indicate that our environment is saturated with chemicals that act like estrogen in our bodies, including BPA. Synthetic estrogens collect in our fat and are more biologically harmful/active than natural estrogens by negatively affecting our DNA.

Phytoestrogens - Plant Estrogens

Virtually everything we eat -- grains, beans, nuts, seeds, seed oils, soy, flaxseed, berries, fruits, roots, vegetables, cabbage, alfalfa and fennel -- contains phytoestrogens. Phytoestrogens change the way estrogen is metabolized by blocking conversion of estrone to dangerous 17B estradiol. They also decrease (down regulate) estrogen receptors (doorways on the cells), thus reducing the amount of estrogen (yours or synthetic) that gets into your cells. Phytoestrogens also stop the production of estradiol by inhibiting the enzyme "aromatase". They also occupy, thus neutralizing, the estrogen receptor sites to prevent harmful estrogens from turning on potentially destructive pathways. This is done by binding to estrogen synthetase, thus inhibiting production of harmful estrogen in the body.

Researchers continue to say mixed phytoestrogens are not harmful at dietary doses! So eat a plant based diet to protect yourself.

Oops? I Just Micro Waved That In Plastic

So you just took out the left overs and put them in the microwave and covered them with plastic wrap. Are you going to die??? Good Housekeeping did a study to see if any BPA/Phthalates leeched into the micro waved food from the plastic. The good news was the products tested contained no phthalates or BPA and they did NOT pick up any after micro waving. Here are the products tested:

Tupperware Crystal Wave lid
Tupperware Rock 'N Serve container
Tupperware Rock 'N Serve lid
Rubbermaid Easy Find Lids lid
Rubbermaid Premier lid
Glad Simply Cooking Microwave Steaming Bags
Ziploc Brand Zip 'n Steam Microwave Steam Cooking Bags
Glad Ware Containers with Interlocking Lids container
Glad Ware Containers with Interlocking Lids lid
Ziploc Brand Containers with Snap 'N Seal Lids container
Ziploc Brand Containers with Snap 'N Seal Lids lid
Webster Industries Good Sense storage container
Webster Industries Good Sense storage container lid
United Plastics 21 oz Bowl
Saran Premium wrap
Saran Cling Plus Clear Plastic Wrap
Glad Cling Wrap Clear Plastic Wrap
Reynolds Clear Seal-Tight Plastic Wrap
Ziploc Brand Storage Bags with Double Zipper
Ziploc Brand Freezer Bags with Double Zipper
Glad Freezer Storage Bags
Reynolds Slow Cooker Liners
Kid Cuisine All Star Chicken Breast Nuggets container
Kid Cuisine All Star Chicken Breast Nuggets film cover
Stouffer's frozen Homestyle Classics Lasagna with Meat & Sauce tray
Stouffer's frozen Homestyle Classics Lasagna with Meat & Sauce film covering Tupperware Crystal Wave container

The following items contained low levels of phthalates or PBA but the chemicals did not leach into the food during microwave heating:

Rubbermaid Easy Find Lids container
Rubbermaid Premier container
Glad Press'n Seal Multipurpose Sealing Wrap
Glad Food Storage Bags

Recycling Number

Many plastic items are marked with a resin ID code, usually a number (1 through 7) or a letter abbreviation, which indicates a particular type of plastic. The code is typically found on the bottom of a container, and is often displayed inside a three-arrow recycling symbol. Resin ID codes are used to help identify different plastics for recycling.

Plastic #1: Polyethylene Terephthalate (PETE)
Common uses: 2 liter soda and juice bottles, cooking oil bottles, peanut butter jars. This is the most widely recycled plastic and often has redemption value under the California "Bottle Bill." #1 plastic contains no BPA, but these bottles contain a potentially carcinogenic element (something called diethylhydroxylamine or DEHA). They are safe for a single use only, but if you must keep them longer, it should be no more **than a few days, a week max, and keep them away from heat as well.**

Plastic #2: High Density Polyethylene (HDPE)
Common uses: detergent bottles, milk jugs, bleach, motor oil, grocery bags, bullet proof vests and yogurt containers. HDPE is the most popular plastic in the world and environmentally friendly.

Plastic #3: Polyvinyl Chloride (PVC)
Common uses: plastic pipes, outdoor furniture, shrink wrap, water bottles, salad dressing and liquid detergent containers.

Plastic #4: Low Density Polyethylene (LDPE)
Common uses: dry cleaning bags, produce bags, trash can liners, food storage containers and trays, play ground slides and six-pack soda can rings. #4 LDPE has more carbon chains than #2 HDPE.

Plastic #5: Polypropylene (PP)
Common uses: bottle caps, drinking straws, ropes, thermal underwear, carpets, laboratory equipment, hernia mesh, surgical suture, loudspeakers, automotive components and stacking chairs. PP resists fatigue, but can break down in UV (sun) exposure. Recycling centers almost never take #5 plastic.

Plastic #6: Polystyrene (PS)
Common uses: packaging pellets or "Styrofoam peanuts," cups, plastic tableware, meat trays, take-out "clam shell" containers. PS breaks down when exposed to acid solutions, such as adding lemon or tomato to foods,

or when food contains vitamin A, or is micro waved. It is a known human neurotoxin and a known animal carcinogen.

Plastic #7: Other

Common uses: certain kinds of food containers, ipod cases, sun glasses, DVDs and Tupperware. This plastic category, as its name of "other" implies, is any plastic other than the named #1-#6 plastic types. These containers can be any of the several different types of plastic polymers. #7 plastic indicates that the plastic may contain BPA, but not always. Recycling centers cannot recycle plastic #7.

Tips For Safety

1. Instead of polycarbonate plastic water bottles, baby bottles etc, use glass, stainless steel or aluminum bottles.

2. When possible, avoid containers that have #7 on the bottom, especially for infants and children. Safe plastics for kids are #1, #2, #4, and #5 which contain no BPA.

3. If you use polycarbonate bottles, don't put hot liquids in them as this releases BPA. Wash these by hand, not in the dishwasher–hot water releases BPA. Don't keep them in the sun or your hot car. Don't put them in the microwave.

4. Opt for food in jars or cartons instead of cans–better to eat fresh/raw or frozen foods. Acidic and fatty foods leech BPA from their cans. If you are feeding a baby, powdered formula is safer than canned liquid formula (unless it states BPA free).

5. Don't reuse plastic water/soda/juice bottles. These have no BPA in them but they may contain bacteria that is impossible to clean out. These bottles, if degraded by repeated washing, dishwasher, or scratches, leech a trace toxic metal antimony.

6. Don't microwave or heat foods in plastic containers. This includes all plastics because when you heat plastic, even if it doesn't contain BPA, heat will release other plastic chemicals that are harmful.

7. The American Chemistry Council reports that phthalates are no longer being used in plastic wraps since 2006. I still would recommend glass containers in the microwave, with glass tops or a paper towel to cover the dish instead of plastic wrap.

* The average American tosses four pounds of trash a day.

**DES was given to pregnant women to prevent miscarriages. It caused an unusual cancer of the reproductive tract in the young women who were exposed in the womb, less so but causing testicular cancer in the men exposed in the womb. Scientists have cataloged a long list of reproductive and other abnormalities linked to DES.

***Estradiol: This is the estrogen correlated with the highest incidence of breast, ovary and uterine cancers.

References:
Williams, F., "Is It Safe To Heat Food In Plastic?," Good Housekeeping.com; 2009
Hunt, P., *"Microwave In Plastic?"* BottomLine.com; 2/1/09:14
"Tough Questions About A Hard Plastic" Wellness Letter, University of California, Berkeley; 25 (5), 2/09:1-2.
Seliger, S., *"BPA:5 Tips To Avoid The Danger In Plastics;"* 2009. http://www.fda.gov/oc/opacom/hottopics/bpa.html
Lang IA, *"Association of Urinary Bisphenol A Concentration With Medical Disorders and Laboratory Abnormalities in Adults"* 2008. http://jama.ama-assn.org/cgi/content/full/300.11.1303.
en.wikipedia.org/wiki/Bisphenol_A
Adlercreutz, H. *"Inhibition of Human Aromatase by Mammalian Lignans and Isoflavonoid Phytoestrogens,"* J Steroid Biochem, 1993; 44:147-153.
Andersson, A., *"Exposure to Exogenous Estrogens in Food. PossibleImpact on Human Development and Health,"* Eur J Endocrin, 1999;140:477-85.
Adlercreutz, H., *"Dietary Phytoestrogens and Cancer: In Vitro and In Vivo Studies,"* J Steroid
Biochem Mol Biol, 1992; 41:331-337.
www.bisphenol-a.org
Hinterthuer, A., *"Just How Harmful Are Bisphenol-A Plastics?"* September 2008; Scientific American Magazine.

CONTROVERSIES IN SOY

Before you:
Eat one more veggie burger
Take one more soy supplement
Drink one more glass of soy milk
What you need to know!

The Joy Of Soy

Soy provides most of our essential amino acids. It is low in fat, is cholesterol free and is an anti-oxidant via isoflavones: genistein anddaidzein. Isoflavones are polyphenolic compounds found in legumes (soy, chickpeas, lentils and beans) and red clover. Saponins in soy enhance the immune function and bind to cholesterol in the gut. Phytosterols in soy lower cholesterol. Soy has phytoestrogenic (plantestrogen) properties. Soy is high in retainable calcium.

Controversies In Soy

Claimed!
"Infants fed soy formula are getting the hormonal equivalent of five birth control pills per day." Daniel Sheehan, Director for the US NationalCenter for Toxicology Research, 1998.

The phytoestrogen in soy has a structure similar to that of regular estrogen: 1/1000th the strength. Soy phytoestrogens do not turn these estrogen receptors on to the same degree as regular estrogen. Genisteinand daidzein bind directly to estrogen receptors (alpha and beta), thus having anti-estrogenic or weak estrogenic effects. Thus, lessening total estrogen effects. There is no progesterone in soy. Therefore, this scary claim is false.

Aluminum

Claimed!

"Soy infant formulas contain high levels of aluminum."

Soybeans are high in aluminum. High aluminum content of the brain has been associated with Alzheimer's disease. The human body absorbs very little aluminum through the bowels and what is absorbed, is excreted by the kidneys, if the kidney function is normal. If you have normal kidney function, you or your child will not have aluminum toxicity from soy products.

Manganese

Claimed!

"Soy formulas cause Manganese Toxicity Syndrome."

Soy formulas can have 50 times more manganese than breast milk. Manganese can be neurotoxic to predisposed babies. It may cause" Manganese-Toxicity Syndrome," which is one of the causes of Attention Deficient Hyperactive Disorder (ADHD). A family in our church must restrict there young son's soy intake to be able to keep him focused. But, in almost all infants and children, it is eliminated from the body without harm.

Protease (Trypsin) Inhibitors

Claimed!

"Protease inhibitors cause cancer in humans."

Protease (trypsin) inhibitors, found in potatoes, eggs, and cereals, is natural soy toxin that can interfere with protein digestion. Researchers have known for years that animals eating raw soybeans failed to grow properly and reproduce, but animals that ate heated or processed soybeans didn't have the same problem. Protease inhibitors are destroyed when processed or cooked. Some have suggested that protease inhibitors may contribute to cancer in humans, but they are actually found to prevent the activation of the specific genes that cause cancer. They also protect against damaging the DNA from radiation and free radicals. Most of the protease inhibitor is destroyed in the preparing of the soy foods we eat, but there may be enough to help lower our cancer risk. Sources of raw soy include soy flour and soy protein concentrate (weightlifting supplements).

Phytic Acid

Phytic Acid (PA), a natural soy toxin, blocks the absorption of Ca, Mg, Zn, and may cause deficiencies in Cu, Fe, Vit.E, K, D and B12. It may cause breast epithelial hyperplasia (an early form of cancer) in mice.

TI, PA and other toxins are reportedly removed by any processing soy undergoes.

38 Beneficial Studies On Soy - The Soy Advantage

1. Fights heart disease-reduces cholesterol by 9-24% (LDL by 5-13% and triglycerides by 10%), and coronary vessels are more flexible. Soy lowers blood pressure, too.

2. Wards off osteoporosis, increases bone density in post menopausal woman. Soy increases tissue vitamin D levels. Substituted soy protein for animal protein decreases urinary calcium excretion.

3. Tames menopausal symptoms in most women, which may have more to do with stress, nutrition and environmental toxin exposure than hormonal balance.

4. May protect against breast cancer. Exposure to soy foods during childhood and adolescence during pubertal breast development provides a unique benefit of reducing breast cancer risk in adulthood. Ann Wu from the University of Southern California showed a 15% reduction in breast cancer risk per serving of tofu, per week.

5. May prevent prostate cancer by blocking conversion to 5-alphadihydrotestosterone (DHT) and fights prostate cancer by slowing growth through genistein.

6. May protect against colon cancer. 50% reduction in polyps-pre cancer.

7. May protect against endometrial cancer.

8. May prevent stroke.

9. Helps prevent diabetic nephropathy (kidney failure).

10. Regulates blood sugar and keeps insulin levels down.

11. Eating soy instead of dairy protein prevents gallstones and even helps dissolves them once formed.

12. Because of its fiber, soy prevents and helps relieve constipation.

13. Soy protects against diverticulosis and hemorrhoids.

14. Soyfoods and isoflavones exert beneficial effects on cognition and memory.

15. Soy acts as an antioxidant/cancer-preventing agent. It inhibits hydrogen peroxide production and superoxide anion generation in cells and can inhibit microsomal lipid peroxidation (cholesterol inflammation).

Soya Say?

How soy helps. As humans age or undergo disease progression, they produce more dangerous cytokines (TNF-a). TNF-a regulates inflammatory genes (NF-kB). Toxic effects of NF-kB include: out of control cancer cell growth, chronic inflammation and auto immune diseases. Soy supplements protect against TNK-a induced activation of NF-kB. Cancer cells often over express NF-kB, making them resistant to normal cell regulation and to the effects of chemotherapy. 12,395 Seventh-day Adventist men who drank soy milk more than once a day were 70% less likely to get prostate cancer. Compared to men in Finland, Portugal and Britain, men in Japan and China have significantly lower risk of prostate disease associated with their higher consumption of isoflavones.

Controversies In Soy

Soy is found in: vitamins, medicines, creams, lotions, rubs, green drinks, baby food, cereal, crackers, milk, soup, cookies, meat substitutes, noodles, hot drinks, sauces, nut substitutes, chips, candy bars, etc. Soy is a drug, like many herbs; so temperance is wise. Some people are allergic to soy protein. It has been suggested that phytoestrogens may stimulate, rather than inhibit, growth of pre-existing, estrogen-dependent tumors. Isoflavones, weak estrogens, when eaten purified, some say, increases your risk for breast CA. (> 100 mg/day). The weight of evidence indicates that, unlike estrogen, soy (even more than 100 mg/day of isoflavones) is not likely to increase breast cancer risk in any women or prostate cancer in men. There is no indication that soy increases clot formation (adversely affecting coagulation and fibrinolytic factors) which could cause stroke, heart attack or pulmonary emboli (clots to the lungs).

Not Soy Fast

Until the 1930s, the only place you could find soybeans was in the local hardware store in paint and varnish. Manufactures must use harsh chemical processing (acid baths and extreme heat) to remove many toxins. Nitrates can be added during the spray drying process. Does this change the protective effects of soy products by the way they are processed compared to other country's forms of processing? I don't know!

Thyroid Interaction And Soy

Soy may cause goiters and hyperthyroidism. (Japan study 1991) Soy binds with the active hormone in Synthroid or like other thyroid supplements and causes faster elimination. Avoid soy for 4 hours after taking your thyroid meds.

Soy What? Unproven But Suggested Soy Effects

Excess estrogen in children can lead to thyroid problems, learning disabilities and premature puberty. In theory: in boys it could increases the risk of testicular cancer and in girls it could increase the risk of breast cancer and ovarian cancer.

If your child has unusual behavioral problems…
If you have asthma or allergic problems…
If you have thyroid problems…
If you have breast tumors or cancer…
If you have stomach ulcers or lack of digestive enzymes…

You may want to moderate your soy products.

Is Soy Really The Problem?

We are exposed to environmental estrogens every day. Is this the reason there are negative reports about soy? Asian study differences, in comparison to American outcomes, may be due to the local plant stress, fungus, growing conditions of the soybean causing it to be anti-estrogen vs. weakly estrogenic. Asians often use highly fermented soy; Americans don't. Soy should not be your only protein, but well balanced, with nuts, legumes and whole grains. Is soy really the problem or artificial estrogens in our midst?

References:

Anderson, JW, *"Meta-analysis Of The Effects Of Soy Protein Intake On Serum Lipids,"* NEJM 1995;333:276-282.

Washburn, S, *"Effects Of Soy Protein Supplementation On Serum Lipoproteins, Blood Pressure, And Menopausal Symptoms In Perimenopausal Women,"* Menopause 1999 Spr;6:7-13.

Wu, A.H., *"Adolescent And Adult Soy Intake and Risk Of Breast Cancer In Asian-Americans,"* Carcinogenesis, 2003; 23(9):1491-1496.

Gaynor, M.L.,*"Isoflavones And The Prevention And Treatment Of Prostate Disease: Is There A Role?"* Cleveland Clinic Journal of Medicine, March 2003; 70(3):203-216.

Anderson, JW, *"Effects Of Soy Protein On Renal Function And Proteinuria In Patients With Type 2 Diabetes,"* Am J Clin Nutr 1998;(suppl):1347S-1353S.

Wei, H, "*Antioxidant And Anti-promotional Effects Of The Soybean Isoflavone Genistein,"* Proc Soc Exp Biol Med 1995;208:124-129.

Messina, MJ, *"Soy Intake And Cancer Risk: A Review Of The In Vitro And In Vivo Data,"* Nutri Cancer 1994;21:113-121.

Jacobsen, B.K., *"Does High Soy Milk Intake Reduce ProstateCancer Incidence? The Adventist Health Study,"* Cancer Causes Control 1998;9:553-557.

File, S.E., *"Eating Soy Improves Human Memory,"* Psychopharmacology, 2001;157:430-436.

File, S.E., *"Improved Memory And frontal Lobe function after 3 months' treatment with soya supplements,"* Eur J Neuropsychopharmacol,2002;12(S3):S406.

Aldercreutz, H, *"Plasma Concentrations Of Phyto-estrogens In Japanese Men,"* Lancet 1993;342:1209-1210.

Lee, HP, *"Dietary Effects On Breast-Cancer Risk In Singapore,"* Lancet 1991;337:1197-2000.

Murkies, AL, *"Dietary Flour Supplement Decreases Post-MenopausalHot Flushes: Effect Of Soy And Wheat,"* Maturitas 1995;21(3):189-195.
Cassidy, A, *"Biological Effects Of A Diet Of Soy Protein Rich Isoflavones On The Menstrual Cycle Of Premenopausal Women,"* Am J Clin Nutr 1994;60:333-340.
Messina, M, *"To Recommend Or Not To Recommend Soy Foods,"* J Am Diet Assoc 1994;94:(11):1253-4.
Div, RL, *"Antithyroid Isoflavones From Soybeans,"* Biochem Pharmacol 1997;54:1087-1096.
Lissin, LW, *"Phytoestrogens And Cardiovascular Health,"* J Am Col Card 2000;35:1403-1410.
Vincent, A, *"Soy Isoflavones: Are They Useful in Menopause?"* MayoClin Proc 2000;75:1174-1184.
Bazzano, LA, *"Legume Consumption And Risk Of Coronary Heart Disease In US Men And Women,"* NHANES I Epidemiologic Follow-up Study, Arch Intern Med 2001;161:2573-2578.
Yildirir, A, *"Soy Protein Diet Significantly Improves Endothelial Functionand Lipid Parameters,"* Clin Cardiol 2001;24:711-716.
A good resource is www.talksoy.com

TYPE D PERSONALITY

- A Risk Factor For Heart Disease

"A merry heart doeth good like a medicine: but a broken spirit drieth the bones." Proverbs 22:17

Solomon must have realized that there are people with un-merry hearts.

What's A Type D Personality?

High levels of worry, irritability, gloom, anger and lack of self assurance are strongly associated with both hypertension and heart disease. Psychiatrists classify the highest distress levels as a "D" type personality (like Eeyore of A.A. Milne's "Winnie the Pooh."). The D type personality is less responsive to treatment and has a poorer quality of life. They are more likely to die prematurely.

The ABC Of Personality

The first attempt to link personality to a medical risk was in the1960s and 1970s. Psychologists devised a short alphabet to describe different tendencies. Type A's, the weekend-working perfectionists, were deemed likely candidates for heart disease. Relaxed, noncompetitive Type B's were supposed to be models of health. And Type C's, outwardly pleasant people who avoided conflict by suppressing their feelings, were said to be cancer-prone. The ABC model for disease and death fell apart in the

1980s when large studies found no reliable connection between the Type A personality and heart disease. Later research has shown that harmful emotions such as anxiety, anger, hostility and hopelessness, are truly life threatening. The D type personality has given researchers an easy way to measure several injurious emotions all at once.

The Results Of The Type D Test

Professor Johan Denollet of Tillburg University, Netherlands (the inventor of this test) found that of the 300 people in the cardiac rehabilitation program given this test (see below), within 10 years 27% of the Type D patients had died of heart disease or stroke, compared to 7 percent of the others. Again, when the Type D questionnaire was given to 875 patients who had recently received coated stents to open their coronary arteries, the type D patients were more than four times more likely than the other patients to experience a heart attack or death within six to nine months after the procedure.

What If You're A Type D Personality?

This isn't a parlor game, but it's worth playing. Don't panic if you score at the high end of the scale. A Type D personality is not a mental illness. It is a collection of normal fallen human traits. Through Christ all inherited and cultivated tendencies to evil can be over come. Do you believe that? A good marriage can be an antidote to social inhibition, especially if your partner's ease with people compensates for your own discomfort. Even the most distress-prone person can learn to cope with stress and beat back anxious thoughts. Many Type D people have trouble seeking help. By definition, they're ill-at-ease and afraid to open up, but family, friends, church family and their physicians can help overcome these barriers.

The Plan For Treatment Of Type D Personalities

Even if you never conquer your distress, you can take practical steps to make it less toxic to your health. Exercise increases your happy hormones in your brain. Eating a diet rich in fresh fruits and vegetables can reduce almost anyone's risk of a heart attack. Lifestyle changes that protect your heart can improve your emotional state. Warding off emotional distress by prayer, Bible study and talk therapy with a friend can help prevent Satan from using your Type D personality to get the best of you.

The Mind Of Satan

"How Satan exults when he is enabled to set the soul into a white heat of anger! A glance, a gesture, an intonation, may be seized upon and used, as the arrow of Satan, to wound and poison the heart that is open to receive it." Our High Calling 235

The Mind Of Christ

"And the multitude of them that believed were of one heart and of one soul." Acts 4:32 *"Every Christian saw in his brother the divine similitude of benevolence and love. One interest prevailed. One object swallowed up all others. All hearts beat in harmony. The only ambition of the believers was to reveal the likeness of Christ's character."* Christ Object Lessons 121

Reference:

The New Frontiers Of Medicine, Harvard Medical School, www.health. harvard.edu, 2006, page 7.

DIABETES

Diabetes And Your Blood Vessels

I explain to all my diabetic patients about diabetes' life threatening risk. Patients with diabetes face the risk of a cardiovascular event. Diabetes increases the risk of premature heart attack and stroke by 10 to 15 years. Heart disease is the primary cause of diabetes-related deaths. Patients with diabetes are two to four times more likely to die of heart and blood vessel disease.

Factors For Early Death

The risk factor of diabetes is equal to the risk factor of coronary heart disease. Coronary heart disease (CHD) occurs when one or more of the coronary arteries that surround the heart become narrower, restricting the flow of blood to the heart muscle. A report from the National Cholesterol Education Program states that diabetes is equal to a CHD risk factor for heart attack and stroke. In addition, individuals with diabetes who experience a heart attack have an unusually high death rate either immediately or in the long term, because the persistently high blood sugar levels effect the rate of hardening of the arteries and disease activity.

Other Complications Of Diabetes

Other complications of diabetes include high blood pressure, blindness, kidney failure, nervous system disease (numb and painful hands and feet), impotence, amputations, dental disease, complications of pregnancy, and is one of many causes of Alzheimer's disease.

References:

Laing,S.P., *"Mortality From Cerebrovascular Disease In A Cohort Of 23,000 Patients With Insulin-Treated Diabetes,"* Stroke, 2003;34:418-421.

Centers For Diseases Control And Prevention Fact Sheet, www.cdc.gov/diabetes/pubs/factsheet.htm.

Facts About Coronary Heart Disease, Washington D.C.:Public Health Service, July 1993, www.nhlbi.nih.gov/health/public/heart/other/chdfacts.htm.

The Third Report Of The National Cholesterol Education Program (NCEP) Expert Panel On Detection, Evaluation, And Treatment Of High Blood Cholesterol In Adults (Adult Treatment Panel III) Executive Summary, NIH, May 2001; NIH Pub No.01-3670.

RELATIONSHIPS

- Kinship With Christ
- Relationship First, Behavior Follows

Your relationship with God reflects your kinship with others--
How you are treated and how you treat them.

Relationship Begats Behavior

Personal relationships involve interactions between fallen, sinful mankind. The success of personal relationships depends upon our outlook on life and the acceptance of individual behavior. Earthly relationships tend to be conditional, which can make it harder to understand our relationship with God, because His involves unconditional love and acceptance. If we don't like the way someone behaves, we may choose not to be friends with them anymore. Because of our sinful tendencies, we often see a very dysfunctional relationship as the only way to have a relationship. But God wants to show us a better way to interact and response to life's stressors. Life's stressors express themselves in how we relate to those around us, through our relationships and our daily behavior. One of the most common comments I receive in my practice of medicine is, "I'm stressed, " in other words "I'm insecure." *"Trust in the Lord with all your heart and lean not unto your own understanding."* Proverbs 3:5

"When the daily experience is one of looking unto Jesus and learning of Him, you will reveal a wholesome, harmonious character." "Words of kindness and sympathy will do as good as a medicine, and will heal souls that are in despair." Gospel Worker, 163.

Dysfunctional Friends And Family

My family is dysfunctional; I am dysfunctional-just ask my wife. We are all dysfunctional to some degree until we get to heaven, but in the mean-time... I have heard it said that no human has psychological problems, only spiritual ones. We cannot affect genuine reform of our characters apart from Christ. Poor relationships are less likely to affect the Christian who is a Christ-like peacemaker. As we grow in our relationship with Christ, we will be able to grow healthy relationships (less dysfunctional) with our friends and family. List two or three of your closest relationships, include yourself. Ask God to show you how you have caused harm in each relationship. This will be very eye opening!

The Book Of Psalms And Our Relationship With God

When I was 18 years old I couldn't understand why God placed the book of Psalms in the Bible. I had no use for it. It was full of emotion and relationships with one's enemies and with God. But by the time I was 30 years old and had a few more life experiences under my belt, I understood why. Psalms is full of good and bad relationships for our example and encouragement.

Resolving Conflict

Behavior defines our "personalities" in the minds of others, and our inherent personalities cause us to behave in certain predictable ways. Conflicts occur daily in our lives. When disagreements and stress (unresolved conflict) reduce the effectiveness of our relationships, it is the responsibility of both parties to facilitate a resolution. Finding the definition of the problem (conflict/stress) is the first step in resolving the conflict. In every situation take hold of the power of prayer, and with earnest, agonizing faith lay hold upon the mighty arm of power (Patriarchs and Prophets, 203). I like to mentally write down what is making me anxious or stressed and pray over these things. Sometimes many times, and sometimes many years. *"The natural co-operates with the supernatural. It is a part of God's plan to grant us, in answer to the prayer of faith, that which He would not bestow did we not thus ask."* Great Controversy, 525

Interpersonal Relationships

1. Do not expect anyone to **be responsible** for your happiness except Christ. Ask yourself why you aren't happy. Too often, relationships fail because someone is unhappy and blames the other person. *"He who is seeking his own glory appeals to the desire for self-exaltation*

in others." Desires of Ages, 212. Being responsible means having the ability to respond, not blame.

2. Make and keep clear agreements. Desire to do the right thing with God's help. **Respect** the differences between yourself and your friend/partner. Do not expect your friend/partner to agree with you on every issue. Love, respect and trust are the cement in any relationship. In humility pray without ceasing. George MacDonald, the eighteenth century Scottish clergyman, said that "to be trusted is a greater compliment than to be loved."
3. Don't expect anybody but God to be able to read your mind. (Are you listening ladies?!) Use **communication** to establish a common ground to understand different points of view. Biblically seek a mutual, collaborative agreement or plan. A true relationship will consist of both parties contributing equally.
4. Approach your relationship as a **learning experience**. Each life lesson has important information for you to learn. Life's bumps can be a witness and testimony during future stress filled events. *"All things work together for good to them that love the Lord."* Romans 8:28 *"It is in crisis that character is revealed."* Christ Object Lessons, 412.
5. **Forgiveness** is a decision of letting go of the past and focusing on the present. It's about taking control of your current situation. If God can forgive you, so can you forgive your brother or sister in life. Christian therapies include prayer about the problem, spiritual journaling, memorization of Bible promises, and following all these with forgiveness. We are commanded in Scripture to forgive. Ephesians 4:32; Colossians 3:13
7. Review your **expectations**. Insecurities are unfulfilled expectations. Worry is a waste of the imagination. Try to be as clear as you can about any expectations-including acceptable and unacceptable behavior and attitudes. Build each other up. Everybody needs agape love and affirmation.

References:

http://two.not2.org/psychosynthesis/articles/rmoore.htm
CQ (Collegiate Quarterly), Pacific Press Pub Ass., 2011:37-45.

MARITAL RELATIONSHIPS
- From A Male Perspective

The emotional differences between males and females are like night and day. A hurting/smart remark or rough play from a male to a male friend would be ignored, while a female could be hurt and offended by it for life.

Why Are Males And Females So Different?

Females want to be treated like royalty (a queen). They want security, closeness, open communication about our (male's) feelings, affirmation (like, 'oh, that looks good on you' or 'that meal was the best,' etc) and tenderness (being treated like a china doll). We males usually don't get it! Thus, we don't supply any of these wants that a female requires to feel secure. From a worldly view, it is said that males give love to get sex and females give sex to get love. Two opposites, yet God wants us to get along. Therefore, we males must try to understand where the female is coming from to survive life together. We must through Christ's help practice patience and understanding without expecting anything in return, even when to us it makes little sense. Sin has made males and females one-sided. We need the other's understanding of life (with each understanding of life very, very different) to be a Christ-like whole-together.

Two Extremes Or One Flesh In Christ?

Females want softness, smells, candles, sweet notes and attention. Males want black and white answers, simple straight forward talk, no strings attached solutions. The failure to understand these two extremes and soften one's approach is one reason many couples break up. This has taken me 25 years to learn and I'm still trying to 'get it.' One can't just admire his mate (mate to be), they must adore them. The spouse is to be another self. The Bible says *'the two should be one'* (Gen 2:24), not which one! "Higher than the highest human joy is the joy God gets whenever a sinner repents and turns to God. And God provides for mankind an earthbound replica in the sexual relationship between husband and wife. As they submit to each other they are fulfilling the love submission symbolism implicit in man's relationship with God." –Today's Youth's Scripture Guide, Quarter 1, Review and Herald; 1977:47.

Service For Others Is The Key To Happiness

To married couples, Ellen White had this to say: *"There should be less display and affection of worldly politeness, and much more tenderness and love, cheerfulness and Christian courtesy, among the members of the household. Many need to learn how to make home attractive, a place of enjoyment. Thankful hearts and kind looks are more valuable than wealth and luxury, and contentment with simple things will make home happy if love be there. God tests and proves us by the common occurrences of life.* ***It is the little attentions, the numerous small incidents and simple courtesies of life, that make up the sum of life's happiness;*** *and it is the neglect of kindly, encouraging, affectionate words, and the little courtesies of life which helps compose the sum of life's wretchedness. It will be found at last that the denial of self for the good and happiness of those around us constitutes a large share of the life record in heaven."* Adventist Home, 108-9.

THINGS I'VE HEARD MY PATIENTS SAY...

Collected by Dr. Royce Bailey over 20 years

Word/Phrase	Meaning	Example
A-fixin'	Getting ready	We're a-fixin to go to the store.
Aim	To intend or to plan	I aim to buy some land. He aims to marry her.
Airish	Cool, breezy or drafty	Shet your window. It's too airish. Hit's getting' right airish out thar.
Askeered of	Frightened or afraid of	He's askeered of his shadow.
Awful poe	Very ill	He's been lookin' awful poe.
Ax	Ask	You ax too many questions.
Belly washer	Large soft drink, ie. Nehi	I'z goin' to the store for a belly washer.
Better than goose grease	Something better than a good thing	That there indoor commode is better than goose grease.

Biggety	Stuck up or acting big	She's been actin' awful biggety these days.
Bile	Boil	The woman had to bile water for the coffee.
Book read	Educated or well informed	We aim for little Flossie to get book read someday.
Bound	Should, must, have to	If ya don't eat, you're bound to git hongry.
Bub	Bulb	The light bub done blowed.
Carry	Transport	Let me carry you to the store.
Carry me	Take me	I'z need you all to carry me to the store.
Cats heads	Biscuits and gravy	Git me some of them there and sopp'ins cat heads and sopp'ins.
Cattywampus	Crooked, as a dog's hind leg	That there road is cattywampus.
Clum'	Climbed	I clum thet hill for the last time.
Conniption fit	Upset and heard by all	She'd throw a conniption fit right there in the parlor.
Cot	To get in trouble	Boy, I cot it when I got home.
Crick	a) A stiffness b) A stream or branch	Marvin has a crick in his neck. I've got runn'in water down at the crick.
Cuttin' up	Acting a fool	Maud shore was cuttin' up last night.
Dast	Dare	Don't you dast ask Zeke to the doin's.
Doin's	A social function	Are you going to the church doin's tonight?
Draws	Spasm or cramp	My leg shore draws.
Et	Eaten	Have you et?
Far	Fire	The far went out and wezin' got cold.
Fetch	To bring	Go fetch the doctor.
Foe	Four	That's the fastest foe legged horse I'd seen.
Fur	Far	That's a fur piece to walk.

Fur piece	A great distance	He lives a fur piece from his kin folks.
Gander	Come look at this!	Do you wanna take a gander at this?
Geet	Have you eaten yet?	Geet? I'm starved!
Gommin'	Loafing and Piddlin'	Why's he a gommin' and a piddlin' instead of a workin'?
Gooch	To poke	Don't gooch me in mayh side
Drownder	A hard rain	That shore was a good drownder last night.
Gully washer	A hard rain	We shore had a gully washer last night.
Hail	Hell	Hail, that hurts.
Hesh up	Become quiet	Make Jess hesh up.
Het	Become heated or upset	Don't let that get you all het up.
Hissie fit	Grip'in, didn't like	I'd throw a hissie fit when I heard it.
Holler	a) a small valley b) yell	She come from over in the holler. Holler at me if you need me.
Hominy	How many	Hominy kids you got?
Jaw	To engage in conversation	Let's jaw a spell.
Keep your	Be prepared	Trust in God and keep your powder dry.
Kindly	Certainly, surely	He kindly has an odor about him.
Kivver	Covered	Them youn-uns is kivvered with the pox.
Lollygag	To loaf, loiter or poke along	Why's Clem always lollygaggin' around?
Mesh	Push	Ya gotta mesh that button.
Mow	More	Gimme some mow of them beans.
Naw	No	Naw, I never fetched the syrup.
Onliest	Only one	He's my oneliest son.
Parts	Area or neighborhood	What's he doin' in these parts?
Pastor	Pasture	The horse is in the pastor.

Peaked	Pale or sick looking	He's lookin' mighty peaked today.
Pizen	Poison	I seen lots a pizen snakes in these parts.
Plum	Completely	I'm plum upset with he rlollygaggin' around.
Plus which	In addition to	We got water in the creek, plus which the well.
Poe	Not rich	I's a poe farmer.
Poke	Paper bag	He put the chicken in a poke.
Put out	Angry, annoyed	He shore was put out 'boutthe meetin'.
Red	To clean or tidy up	Red up your room.
Runt	No longer of value	You put too much salt in the soup and now hits runt.
Shed of	Get rid of or unload	You got to get shed of that old mule.
Skittish	Nervous	Them mules get kinda skittish when his dogs howl.
Slicker than than owl s...t	Really slippery	That wet hillside is slicker owl s...t (snoot)
Smack-dab	on the spot exactly	I shot him smack-dab through the heart. Hit landed smack-dab on my toe. toe.
Smart	To hurt	It shore smarts where I got hit.
Spell	A period of time	Come set a spell.
Suwannee	Swear	Well, I Suwannee.
Tar	Tire	I cain't go 'cause I got a flat tar.
Tore up	Emotionally upset	I'z all tore up about the barnburnin'.
Tuck	Past tense of take	I ain't tuck a drink this week.
Vittles	Food or Victuals	I hope Ma's got the vittles on when I git home.
Whupped	Whipped or spanked	Pa shore whupped me when ifibbed to the widow women.
You'ns	You or you all	You'ns ain't going to get no vittles.

Doctor-Ease

Word/Phrase	Meaning	Example
A day and night	24 hours	I don't smoke much – not a night more'n a pack in a day and night.
A week to die sudden	Real slow	I'm so slow it'll take me a week to die sudden.
Achanch	Chance	He's taking a achanch.
Afar	A fire	He came from a-far at Jed's place.
Arthur	Arthritis	Old Arthur got me bad. Got somp'n for it?
Bad for	Infamous for	He's bad for burping inpublic.
Can't make a branch.	Can't urinate (pee)	I gotta go and can't make a branch.
Clumb	Climbed	He club up that there pole jes' as neat as a cat
Cures all, kills none.	Good doctor	He's a good doctor, cures all, kills none.
Dead pig in the sunshine	In bliss	I'm happy as a dead pig in the sunshine.
Diddlee squat	Worth nothing	That there new medicine you gaves me sworth diddlee squat.
Down to the short rows	Nearly done	Recon we're down to the short rows – only 20 charts left.
Duck-legged	Bow-legged	Her mama was kinda duck-legged.
Everwho	Whoever	Ever who talked to me was real mean.
Fat chance	Very unlikely it will happen	Fat chance you'll take Nelly to the dance.
Fireballs of the Eucharist	Fibroids of the uterus	I had my fireballs of the Eucharist took out.
Get shed of	Get rid of	I need to get shed of that man. He's a pure drunk.
Good to go	Ready and waiting	Your car's good to go for that Missouri trip.

Head knockerover	Strong force	Him dying was a real headknockerover.
Head screwed on straight	Not crazy	He's got to have his head screwed on straight to be datin' my daughter.
I ain't lyin'	I'm lying	I ain't lyin, he's bigger'n a house.
Ill as a red-tailed wasp	Extremely irritable	She's ill as a red-tailed wasp since her divorce.
In high cotton	Doing well financially	We were in high cotton after we got that van.
In moveable	Doing ok	I was in moveable health till health this here stroke jumped on me.
Jittery as a paint shaker	Nervous	That medicine made me jittery as a paint shaker.
Kidneys acted	Urinated	My kidneys hain't acted in two days.
Knocked me a-whining	Hit me hard	When I complained, Pa knocked me a-whining.
Long on drywall short on studs	Not well put together	That cashier is long on drywall and short on studs.
Mash	Press	Mash on that gas pedal, honey, we're outa here!
My feel bad's hurtin'	Don't feel good	Doc, my feel bad's hurtin' all over.
Nervous as a chicken	Agitated, anxious and irritable	She was as nervous as a chicken, but that Valium holp her.
Nose out of joint	Upset	Don't get your nose out of joint over it.
Pin stroke	Mini stroke (Transient IschemicAttack)	Pa'd been having these pin strokes, but now it's the big one.
Powerful	Deeply moved	You'n made me powerful happy
Pyurt	Well, energetic	I feel right pyurt today.
Real puny	Very sick	She's been real puny since her surgery.
Reck'n	To consider	I reck'n I'd better get overto Klim's 'bout now.

Right smart	Wise	That there was right smart of them city folks to leave.
Scowers	Diarrhea	He's been vomiking and got the scowers to boot.
Slim chance	Doubtful it will happen	There's a slim chance of rain.
Smooth as Ex-Lax	Real easy-like	The trip to town went smooth as Ex-Lax.
Swimmy-headed	Dizzy	After taking that 'ere medicine, I got right swimmy- headed.
Thumpin' gizzard	Heart	Well, bless my little thumpin' gizzard.
Tore all to pieces	Emotional upset	I is tore all to pieces 'cause my uncle died.
Toucheous	Painful to touch	Ow! That spot there's a mighty toucheous.
Traveling fart	Lots of migrating belly gas pain	She had her a traveling fart, but that Mylanta holp her go.
Weak as strained cat pee	Weak, washed out	Doc, I'm weak as strained cat pee.

THE TOP TEN PREDICTIONS FOR THE NEW YEAR

1. The Bible will still have all the answers.
2. Prayer will still work.
3. The Holy Spirit will still move.
4. God will still inhabit the praises of his people.
5. There will still be God-anointed preaching.
6. There will still be singing of praise.
7. God will still pour out blessings upon his people.
8. There will still be room at the cross.
9. Jesus will still love you.
10. Jesus will still save the lost.

THE SOMETIMES FUN PARENT'S OLYMPICS

"Wherefore seeing we also are compassed about with so great a cloud of witnesses, let us lay aside every weight, and the sin which doth so easily beset us, and let us run with patience the race that is set before us," Heb. 12:1

Boxing--to see if the parent or caregiver can pick up the zillion ABC blocks, Lincoln Logs, Legos and Tinkertoys scattered across the floor, under and behind the furniture and place them in the correct boxes before the child takes them out again.

Wrestling--bedtime. To see if your child can fall asleep before the parent does! The child is: changed again (seems like the eightieth diaper today), taken to the toilet again (potty training one hundredth time), read worship story, gotten two drinks of water, taught the memory verse, turning on all the music boxes (do the stores have any left?), rocked in their chair and sung songs. The parent is almost asleep and the child is wide awake----still. So we read the story again, potty again (child states they "forgot". They only went 5 minutes ago!), drink again, say memory verse again. Now the parent is sound asleep until the child jumps on their stomach.

Triathlon:

Event 1--carry tricycle three blocks, (child insisted on bringing it, now refuses to ride it), then across at least three lanes of traffic in each direction–with the mother holding one arm of 3 year old (child refuses to hold hand), with another arm holding the trike, and the other hand pushing the toddler in a stroller. (It's a triathlon-the Lord will provide a way!)

Event 2--running: the family is late for church with the children buckled into their car seats crying, the husband revving the engine of the car in the drive way and the mother sprinting back to the second floor of the house four separate times for: 1) child's security blanket, 2) four more diapers, "just in case", 3) the labels for sabbath school and 4) the offering left out on the counter so it would not be forgotten. The mother that arrives to church most composed wins.

Event 3--swimming: points for: 1) squeezing into the bathing suit that won't cause the neighbors to move away. Wearing old maternity suit doesn't count. 2) being able to stay dry by jumping between splashes, 3) continuing to blow up the inflatable toys until you faint, 4) properly removing a resistant child from the pool because of change in skin color (when normal skin tone changes to sky blue).

"Hi" jump--preliminary warmup: parents engage in some loving exercises. Event: from out of nowhere the 3 year old (who is sucking a thumb and carrying a blanket and at late check was sound asleep) appears at the side of your bed and says "hi". Points for height of parent's horizontal jump. There are no points for the creative explanation given to the child.

Broad Jump--able to leap from the ground floor to the third step of the stairs in a single bound, with a child in one arm, over the following obstacles waiting to go up the stairs: two baskets of clean laundry and hangers, the vacuum cleaner, cleaned-out potty chair, emptied trash baskets, unopened bills to be paid and assorted toys.

Soccer (sock-her)--this event tries the caregiver's patience by seeing how many times: 1) the older child can hit the younger child without being detected, 2) the younger child can take away the older child's security blanket without getting hit and 3) the loud blood curdling cries have broken the precious silence of the last 15 seconds.

Basketball--given a laundry basket full of socks, entrant must match the pairs (same size, make and color), roll them into balls and toss them into the proper drawers. This event may be impossible to win because 1) husbands have never been known to attempt this, 2) husbands that do, claim they are color blind, and 3) nobody can find the mate to every sock (I think the wash machine eats them!).*

"The Saviour regards with infinite tenderness the souls whom he has purchased with his blood. They are the claim of His love. He looks upon them with unutterable longing. His heart is drawn out, not only to the best trained and most attractive children, but to those who by inheritance and through neglect have objectionable traits of character. Many parents do not understand how much they are responsible for these traits in their children. They have not the tenderness and wisdom to deal with the erring ones whom they have made what they are. But Jesus looks upon these children with pity. He traces from cause to effect.

The Christian worker may be Christ's agent in drawing these faulty and erring ones to the Saviour. By wisdom and tact he may bind them to his heart, he may give courage and hope, and through the grace of Christ may see them transformed in character, ..." Ministry of Healing-1905, p 44. (While reviewing this article with several hospital staff members, Candice Crouch our dietitian at Park Ridge Hospital suggested this beautiful quote.)

"... suffer little children, and forbid them not, to come unto me: for such is the kingdom of heaven." Matt 19:14

"Blessed are the meek, for they shall inherit the earth." Matt 5:5

Dedicated to the selfless work of all caregivers-from Royce and Judy Bailey.

* expanded from "The Mom's Olympics" by Jane Mackay, women's day 8/11/92, p 146.

THINK POSITIVE

That dreaded word NO. Often equated with the rules of the church—"NO! You can't do this," or "NO! You can't do that." How would Christ have dealt with each situation when NO or saying something worse is the easiest answer available?

We said BC (Before Children) that we would never do the things we disliked about how our parents raised us but we have found (surprising to us) the same words coming out of our mouths, including NO. "NO, you can't eat in-between meals, you should have eaten more for breakfast." "NO, you can't stand up on the kitchen table." "NO, you must sit here until we are finished with worship." "NO, you must not throw your peas on the floor when we have asked you to clean your plate." "NO, you may not take your dress off during church." "NO, you can not draw on the wall with that red magic marker." We have come to hate this word due to our own overuse.

What seems to achieve positive results more quickly is re-enforcing the good behavior which is desired. We recently knelt down to have worship and prayer and Jillionna (2 1/2 yrs.) decided she was going to test our authority by heading the opposite direction with her baby buggy. Josianne at the same time was quietly kneeling with her tiny hands folded showing reverence to God. (We are still working on closed eyes during prayer). By praising Josianne's good behavior, Jillionna quickly returned, knelt down and folded her hands to receive the same parental approval. No one had to reprimand and say that dreaded word NO. This has worked consistently (as long as we remember to us it).

This same approach can work with adults in the grocery store, bank line and other frustrating situations by looking for the positive. We have found it opens the door to conversion and friendship instead of strife (Proverbs 9:7-9, 10:18-21, 11:9, 12:14, 15:1-2). Christ surely encourages the positive in us and we should strive to emulate this in our daily walk with HIM.

MAKE A SCENE OR MAKE A MEMORY

Considering a 1 1/2 and 2 1/2 year old live in our house, as family life directors, we thought that sharing one of Judy's recent days could illustrate how children teach us about God.

--*"merciful...gracious, slow to anger."* Ps 103:8.

The day was going quite well; it was only 8:30 AM. Wanting to rehearse for an upcoming concert I sat down to practice the harp. Half way through the first song (ten in all), I noticed that no babbling, laughter, or giggles were coming from the room in which the children were playing. I got up to investigate. Much to my horror the kitchen and family room were filled with a cloud of white substance; yes a 10 pound bag of flour covered the floor and filled the air. Jillee and Josee looked like they had been hit by a snow storm, as did the house. My immediate thought was to_______(cannot be printed) and then I remembered a thought from a book I read (pre-children), "Make a scene or make a memory." Mustering up a few ounces of control, I fished for the camera through my flour-dusted contact lenses. "Snap" went the camera, and I had made a memory. Back to the harp for more practice and another quiet moment surfaced. This time my children were making onion soup on their play stove that Grandma had given them for Christmas. Yes, with real onions. They first peeled the onions, leaving them all over the kitchen and family room floor, then placed some of them in their play pots to cook on their stove until "tender," just like mommy. I had already vacuumed the floor twice that morning, once after breakfast and again after the flour tornado, and it was only 9:00 AM. I thought certainly this time I could make a scene and teach these children a lesson but that book, "Make a Scene or Make a Memory," haunted my soul. "Snap" went the camera, whoosh went the vacuum and it was back to the harp. Several songs later you guessed it, that dreaded silence which revealed a floor and sofa sprinkled with bits and pieces of uncooked 'Top-Ramen' soup noodles. Two little faces smiled with glee when my eyes fell upon this mess. How could I make a scene? "Snap" went the camera, whoosh went the vacuum and yes, this "Make a Memory" gets to be expensive film-wise but will be well worth the investment in memories and emotions life years to come. Ecclesiastes 7:9

PS The cupboard housing the above products has been childproofed.

CHILD RULES

Susannah Wesley had nineteen children, including John (the famous preacher) and Charles (the famous hymn writer). To manage her very large family successfully, she followed these rules:

1. Eating between meals is not allowed.
2. Children are to be in bed by 8 p.m.
3. They must take medicine without complaining.
4. Teach a child to pray as soon as he can speak.
5. Require all to be still during family worship.
6. Give them nothing they cry for, and only that which they ask for politely.
7. To prevent lying, punish no fault which is first confessed and repented.
8. Never punish a child twice for a single offense.
9. Commend and reward good behavior.
10. Never allow a sinful act to go unpunished.
11. Any attempt to please, even if poorly performed, should be commended.
12. Preserve property rights, even the smallest matters.
13. Strictly observe all promises.
14. Require no daughter to work before she can read well.
15. Teach children to fear the Lord.
16. Subdue self-will in a child, and thus work together with God to save the child's soul.

As all mothers today, Mrs. Wesley was concerned with the physical, mental, spiritual, emotional growth of her children. Not even today's child psychologist experts could improve on these rules she used nearly 300 years ago. In the Biblical story of Hannah and Samuel: *"For this whole life shall he be given over to the Lord."* 1 Sam. 1:28

BAILEY'S Green Drink

Place in your Blender:

- One handful of: roughly chopped fresh spinach (can get pre-packaged in vegetable isle of grocery store). We sometimes change to other greens-Kale, Collards, etc. We've added 1/2 a bunch of cilantro for more detoxifying effect, but this changes the taste a lot!
- 1/2 inch slice of raw ginger root
- One stalk of celery
- Juice squeezed from 1/2 lime
- Fruit-we've used any of these in combination: mango, apple, peach, banana (fresh or frozen), etc.
- One cup water

Blend and drink. Use fresh because the drink loses its antioxidant effect if not consumed right away.

BLUE RIBBONS FOR GOD

"Hurry up, Royce. Your mare will be stiff as a board after standing in her stall all day. You just can't seem to do anything right and now your class is being called."

Carol was always right there with the criticisms and verbal jabs. Tonight I just didn't need her strident voice to remind me that I was indeed 'way behind schedule in getting my mare ready for the show ring and the three classes in which I was to ride. I had worked hard to prepare Suzy for these Western Performance classes and I knew that my days of riding in the show ring were almost over. My life was getting busier and busier with college classes and soon I would be leaving for my long anticipated year as a student missionary in Kenya, East Africa. These hours of working with my mare were especially precious.

But Suzy was known as a Sabbath-keeping quarter-horse, as I am a Sabbath-keeper. She did not attend shows on the Bible Sabbath, sometimes losing valuable and hard worked-for points which would qualify me for a year-end championship. She did not practice on Sabbath either, nor travel to and from the show on the 7th Day. It took planning, of course, but my resolution was positive. Sometimes it was a tight schedule, as it was tonight, when the sun set late in the overheated summer sky and I knew that the horse show would be well on its way even before I set foot on the fair grounds.

I had placed all my equipment in my car on Friday afternoon, with my boots polished, chaps, saddle and bridle all shined and organized. Suzy had been hauled to the fair grounds on Friday afternoon so that I would have a two hour practice with her after my last college lab. Then she was blanketed and put into her stall for the twenty-four hour Sabbath.

Suzy was waiting for me; she had caught the excitement of the fair with its sounds and smells and she almost leaped from her stall as I put the halter over her ears. It was here that Carol caught me with her insistence that I hurry. How could she understand that sundown worship must be concluded before I even started for the show and that the edges of the Sabbath are just as dear and important as the heart of it?

Now, I patted Suzy's soft nose, white, gentle and eager, as I tightened the cinch and swung into the saddle. We trotted out to the show ring with Carol's admonitions ringing in my ears. She had been right. There had been no time to practice and Suzy was stiff, well into the bit, with her nose too far forward and head held far too high. I had to use too much rein and too much leg to keep her gait easy and slow. It takes a good warm-up before every show performance to remind these Western horses that a loose and easy walk, jog and lope is essential for a high point performance.

My first class of the evening was Western Pleasure and the judges look for the horse with the most ease of motion, one that is completely off the bit and taking each gait with a relaxation that is almost sleepy. The horse that lopes too fast, or the one that requires too much of the rider's hand on the reins is not the one to receive the blue ribbon.

As we jogged along the white rail fence I could feel the judges eyes on me. I watched Carol's black gelding, so slow and easy ahead of me, go into a perfect lope with little restraint, taking exact leads and giving an excellent performance. I asked Suzy for the same easy motion but she was to high, too eager and into the bridle so much that my hands shook. We did the best we could but I knew our number would not be called at the line-up time.

Fortunately we had time in the practice ring before the next two classes of the evening. Carol, who had indeed been given a ribbon during the last class, sniffed audibly as she whirled past me.

"Told you so! When will you learn that horses have to be worked hard before you take them into the show ring? You should have been out here all day, like I was!"

The last class of the evening was Western Riding. The horses were asked to respond to the command of the rider through and over several prescribed obstacles, all duplicating what a well trained horse might be required to do on a working cattle ranch. The horse is never to break stride, never to resist any of the patterns and to keep that loose, easy, controlled gait that represents consummate skill and hard work. Suzy and I had prepared diligently but I knew that many fine horses would be in that ring along with us.

Suzy entered the ring smoothly and we jogged through the large wire gate. She turned to let me fasten and twist the handles and then, obligingly, backed slowly so that I could shut the hinges firmly. The bleachers were filled and an audible hush hung over the whole ring. I could see the judges checking off my "gate entry". I urged Suzy into a lazy lope and we executed the figure eight, changing leads several times and following the patterns in the middle of the arena. Then it was time for the obstacles and the running slide. I leaned over to check Suzy's bit and the heat of her body made me realize what exertion she had made for me and what tension we both felt. Suzy caught my emotion and she put her great heart into one supreme effort. I could feel her muscles lunge under me and I knew she was responding, not only to the love we shared, but to her training. She took the bit softly, tucked her beautiful head, brought those long white legs into perfect symmetry and slide half way down the ring. The crowd went wild and shouted and clapped their approval. I could hear my name called among the clapping and the sound was good. At the line-up time, when all twenty-six riders presented their horses to the judges, Suzy turned her head as if to look at me and I could almost see her wink. She was a good old mare.

I was elated to have done my best and I did receive the blue ribbon that night. As I hung the ribbon in the truck window, in preparation for taking Suzy back home, I mused about being God's trophies here on earth. With preparation, sacrifice, and determination we can all be God's peculiar people and win that most handsome and wonderful gift He offers to all of us . . . . Eternal Salvation.

Written during Royce's Second Year at La Sierra University-Southern California. Occurring at the Nation's Largest County Fair-Los Angeles. Royce Bailey M.D., M.P.H., F.A.A.C., M.A.A.C. is a graduate of Loma Linda University and is currently Medical Director of Cardiology Services at Park Ridge Health, Fletcher, N.C.-Adventist Health Systems.

About Doctor Bailey

Dr. Bailey was born and raised in Los Angeles, California. He received his medical school education and training at Loma Linda University, in Southern California. His medical experience includes two trips to Saudi Arabia with the nationally acclaimed Heart Team from Loma Linda University. He has shared his skills and Christian experience with schools in Kenya, Africa where he spent a year as a student missionary.

After completing his specialty training in Cardiology, he and his wife, Judy, moved to Fletcher, North Carolina to begin his practice at Park Ridge Health, Adventist Health System. He is currently Director of Cardiac Services, and has served as Chief of Staff and Director of the Intensive Care Unit.

He is a Crohn's Disease survivor. For over 30 years he has been active with community health lectures and programs in the areas of cholesterol, lipids, dietary habits, early aging and the decreased immune response from the average diet. He has shared his expertise with groups such as AARP, church lecture programs of various faiths, Rotary Clubs and camp meeting series.

In his spare time he tours with his wife and two daughters (15 time Angel Award Winner) as they Praise the Lord with their harps and other musical instruments.

He also enjoys sharing his love of the Lord with local churches.